Health & Social Care
for GCSE

Mark Walsh

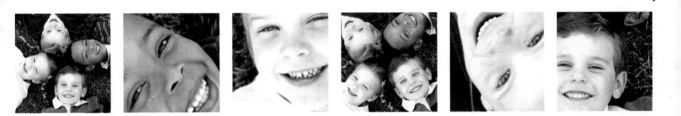

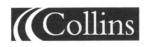

CONTENTS

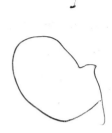

UNIT 3 UNDERSTANDING PERSONAL DEVELOPMENT AND RELATIONSHIPS 150

Acknowledgements

For Karen

Thanks are due to everyone who provided the
help, support and hard work needed to get this
book completed
Mark Walsh

The author and publisher would like to thank the
following for permission to reproduce photographs
and other material:

Barnardo's: logo p. 40
Bubbles: *Dr Hercules Robinson* pp. 9 [centre], 79
[centre left]; *Lois Joy Thurston* p. 38; *Angela
Hampton* p. 49 [top right]; *Jennie Woodcock* p. 66
[bottom], *Pauline Cutler* p. 67 [top]
BUPA: p. 42
Commission for Racial Equality: p. 77
Dogs for the Disabled: p. 41
Ealing, Hammersmith & Hounslow
  Primary Care Trust: p. 51
Belinda Evans: illustrations p10, p.45
Format: *Joanne O'Brien* pp. 9 [bottom left], 57 [top
right], 59, 79 [middle left], 64, 74, 194; *Sally
Lancaster* p. 32; *Paula Stolloway* pp. 15, 57
[bottom left], 69 [bottom], 79 [centre right], 80;
Mo Wilson p. 17; *Maggie Murray* pp. 43, 151
[centre left], 164 [bottom left]; *Brenda Prince*
pp. 44, 61, 76 [left]; *Jacky Chapman* p. 60; *Miriam
Reik* pp. 84 [centre], 131
Health Education Authority: pp. 85 [top left], 98,
106, 114, 117 [top], 137, 143, 144
Helen Evans: pp. 57 [bottom centre], 65, 84
[bottom left], 100 [bottom], 198, 216
Helen Lewis: p. 34 [top]
Hulton Archive; pp. 157 [centre], 215
Jay Ward: p. 94 [centre]
J Mannion: p. 49 [left]
Joseph Rowntree Foundation: p. 40
Kay Wright: pp. 14 [top], 22 [top left], 33, 100
[top], 118, 136, 140, 141, 150 [bottom], 199, 211
Mark Walsh: pp. 34 [bottom], 35 [both], 37, 41,
82, 92, 93, 105, 108, 138, 148, 121, 176, 178.
Mary Evans Picture Library: p. 91
Mike Watson: pp. 22 [top right], 87, 122, 182
[top].
Wendi Watson: p. 189
Mother & Baby Picture Library: pp. 151 [centre
right], 164 [top left & right, bottom right]

NHS Careers: p. 60 [top]
NSPCC: logo p. 40
Olga Mundy: pp. 151 [centre right], 210
Patricia Briggs: pp. 95 [bottom], 105
Phil Read: p. 18
Photofusion: *Bob Watkins* pp. 160, 162, 180, 181;
Paul Baldesare p. 79 [top left], 151 [bottom], 191;
Sam Tanner p. 183; *Steve Eason* p. 204; *Clarissa
Leahy* pp. 168, 169
Popperfoto: p.30
Powerstock/Zefa: p.20
Roger Scruton: p. 182 [bottom]
RoSPA: p. 108
Royal College of Nursing Photo Library: p. 81
Sally Boothroyd: pp. 9 [bottom left], p. 19
S&R Greenhill: *Richard Greenhill* pp. 21, 27, 48
[right], 62, 69 [top], 76, 102 [top], 104, 151 [top
left], 197; *Sally Greenhill* pp. 8 [bottom], 11, 14
[both], 23 [top], 25, 48 [left], 49 [bottom right], 57
[top left], 57 [bottom right], 68 [bottom], 59, 66
[top], 68 [top & centre], 70, 72, 79 [top both] &
bottom left], 84 [top], 85 [bottom right], 94 [top],
101, 116, 129, 123, 127, 128, 129, 188 [right],
191; *Kaye Mayers* p. 188 [left]; *Sam Greenhill*
pp. 172, 208
Science Photo Library: pp. 85 [top right], 88, 115,
120, 186; *Mark Clarke* pp. 85 [centre right], 133;
Ruth Jenkinson p. 135
SCOPE: logo p. 29
Sylvia Kwan: pp. 9 [top right], 16 [top left]
Tim Walsh: pp. 167, 214
Wellcome Photo Library: p. 24, 89, 90, 95 [top &
centre]; *Fiona Pragoff* pp. 23 [bottom], 67 [bottom];
Anthea Sieveking pp. 8 [top & centre], 13, 16
[bottom], 53, 85 [bottom right], 95 [centre], 102
[bottom], 150 [top], 156, 157 [top], 192
World Health Organisation: logo p. 87

Every effort has been made to contact copyright
holders, but if any have been inadvertently
overlooked, the publishers will be pleased to make
the necessary arrangements at the first opportunity.

The purpose of this book

The purpose of this book is to help you to develop the knowledge and understanding that you'll need to complete a GCSE Health and Social Care course. The book has been written specifically to cover the topics in each of the three units that make up your GCSE course.

GCSE Health and Social Care units

Unit 1   Health, social care and early years provision

Unit 2   Promoting health and wellbeing

Unit 3   Understanding personal development and relationships

I've tried to write a book that helps you to gain a good, clear understanding of a range of care topics and also gives you a taste of what to expect from a career in the health and social care sector. Taking a GCSE Health and Social Care course gives you an opportunity to decide whether this is an area of work that you are suitable for and interested in pursuing. Hopefully, you'll think about taking your interest in health and social care further when you've worked through the book and completed your GCSE.

How does the book work?

The book is organised in the same way as your GCSE Health and Social Care course. There are three main units and these are divided into double-page topics. For example, the topic 'Care needs of children' is covered on page 16 and 17. The topics covered in each unit are listed on the contents page at the start of the unit. You can also find the topics that you're looking for by using the index at the end of the book.

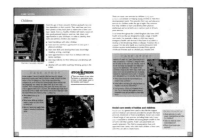

Every double-page topic spread has a number of features. These include the topic information as well as Case Study, Stop and Think and Quick Question activities. You should try to complete the activities as you come to them because they are designed to help you to learn and understand the topic information more clearly. Each of the units also includes four or five pages called Build Your Learning. These provide you with an opportunity to revise what you know and to test your understanding of the topics that you should have learnt about. Completing the activities and the Build Your Learning pages won't always be easy, but it will help you to learn more. It's worth making the effort if you want to achieve the best grade that you're capable of.

What is different about this GCSE?

GCSE Health and Social Care is a **vocational qualification.** This means that it is work-related. It aims to provide the basic knowledge, skills and understanding that you will be able to use in a care workplace or as the basis for further education or training in this area. The content of the course and the work that you do will all be related to the health and social care area in some way. For example, you'll look at the types of care services that exist in the United Kingdom, and the range of care practitioners who provide these services, explore how different behaviours, such as smoking cigarettes and taking regular exercise, affect personal health, and investigate the ways human beings grow and develop throughout life. This means that all of the topics you cover will be related to people who use or provide care services and to the ways that these services are organised and run.

What will my GCSE Health and Social Care cover?

All GCSEs in vocational subjects are composed of three compulsory units. The titles and general focus of your three compulsory units are set out below.

GCSE Health and Social Care units	
Unit title	**What's it about?**
1. Health, social care and early years provision	The types of care organisations that exist, the services they provide, the care workers who work in them, and the skills they need to do so.
2. Promoting health and wellbeing	What 'health' means, factors that have a positive effect on health, factors that damage health, ways of measuring physical health and ways of promoting health improvement.
3. Understanding personal development and relationships	The patterns of growth and development that human beings experience, factors that affect growth and development and the effects of life events and relationships on personal development.

Your teacher will have a course specification that sets out each unit content in detail. You may be given a copy at the start of your course.

How will my GCSE Health and Social Care course be assessed?

GCSE Health and Social Care requires you to work at the same level as any other non-vocational GCSE, such as history or mathematics. The qualification that you'll receive when you complete the course will be graded on an A* to G scale. However, GCSE Health and Social Care is a double award. This means that you will receive the equivalent of two GCSEs at the grade you are awarded when you complete the course. Your grade will therefore be somewhere between A*A* and GG.

To gain a graded GCSE qualification you will need to complete an assessment of your learning in each of the three course units. You will have to complete assignments set by your teachers for units 1 and 2 and you must also sit a test set by the Awarding Body (examination board) for unit 3. You will need to complete each of these three assessments to gain a GCSE Health and Social Care award.

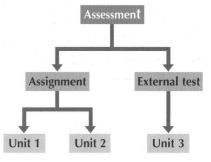

What can I do with my GCSE Health and Social Care?

A GCSE Health and Social Care qualification can help you progress into further education, training or employment. For example, alongside other GCSEs, your health and social care qualification could give you access to AS and A level courses at your school or at a local college, or you may prefer to use it to gain entry to a BTEC First or National course in a vocational area such as care or child care. Alternatively, a GCSE Health and Social Care qualification could help you to obtain a Modern Apprenticeship or an NVQ training course in health, social care or child care. A third option could be to use your GCSE Health and Social Care award to gain employment as a support worker or trainee carer.

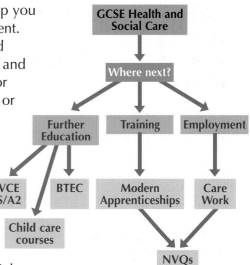

Whatever your career plans, a GCSE Health and Social Care course should provide you with an opportunity to explore and develop your knowledge and understanding of this interesting vocational area. I hope that this is an enjoyable experience and that the book is useful in helping you to achieve the best grade that you're able to.

ealth, social care and early years provision

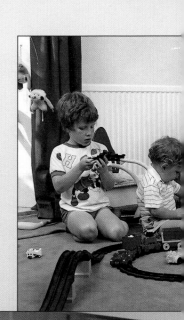

This unit is about care services. You will learn about:

- the care needs of different client groups
- the different types of care services provided for each client group
- the ways care services are organised
- ways of obtaining care services
- the reasons people sometimes don't get the care services that they need
- the jobs and skills of people who work in health, social care and early years organisations
- the values, or ideas, that care workers put into practice when they care for their clients.

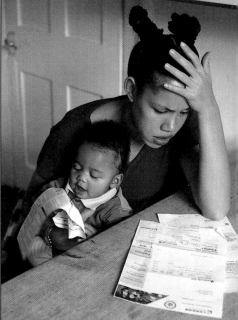

If you are thinking about working in the health, social care or early years system, studying this unit will help you to develop a good understanding of how the care system works and the different jobs that are available within it. If you have another type of career in mind, you can still benefit from studying this unit. Finding out how the care system works will improve your chances of obtaining the care that you or members of your family may need in the future.

Unit 1 of this book covers Unit 1, Health, social care and early years provision, of the GCSE Health and Social Care award.

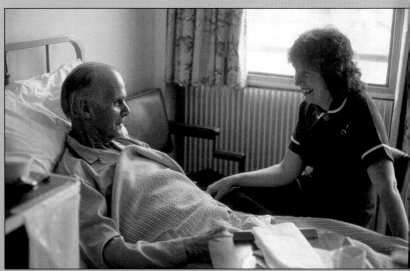

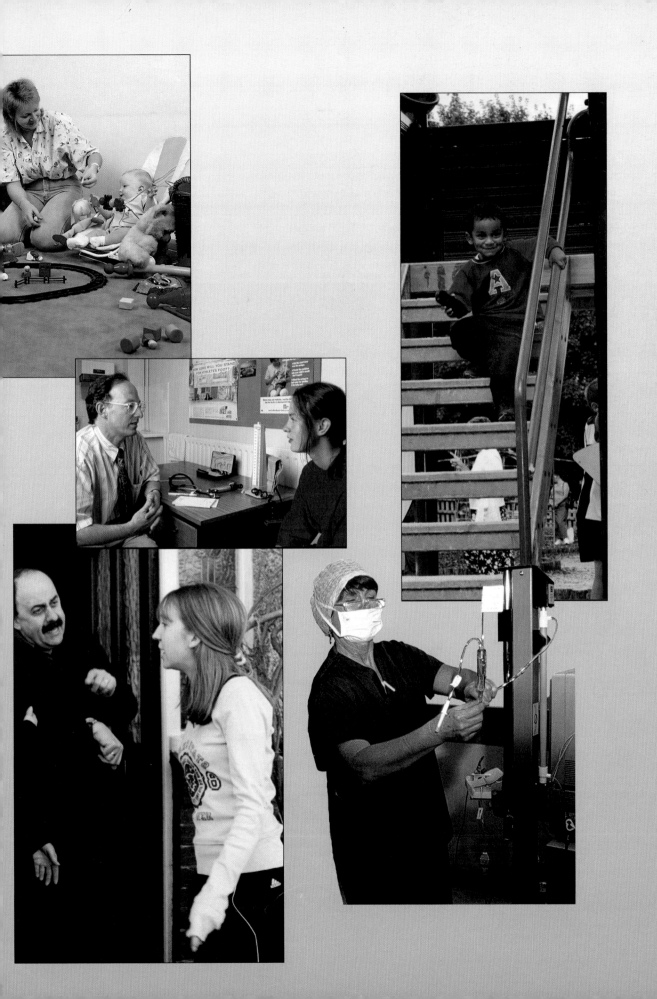

Basic needs and care

To be healthy and feel good about life a person must be able to meet his or her basic needs. **Basic needs** are the things that all human beings require to survive and develop. For example, human beings have a basic physical need for food and drink, shelter and warmth. There are many reasons why a person may not be able to meet their basic needs at different points in their life. For example, a life-threatening injury, too much stress or not having enough money for food, warm clothing or shelter can all lead to health and personal problems.

As well as having physical needs, people have intellectual, social and emotional needs.

- Intellectual needs – to learn about and understand themselves and the world in order to develop and live a fulfilling life.
- Social needs – for relationships and contact with other people.
- Emotional needs – for love and affection, trust, and emotional bonds with family, friends and colleagues.

A person has **unmet needs** when they are unable to obtain the things that they require for survival, good health or development.

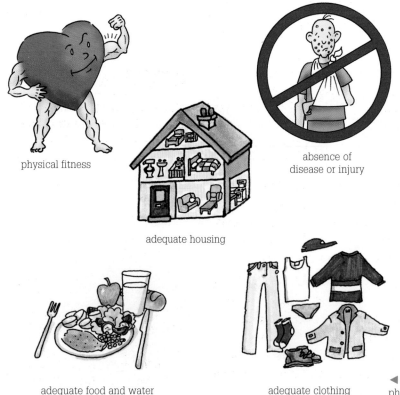

physical fitness

absence of
disease or injury

adequate housing

adequate food and water

adequate clothing

◄ Examples of the basic
physical needs we all have

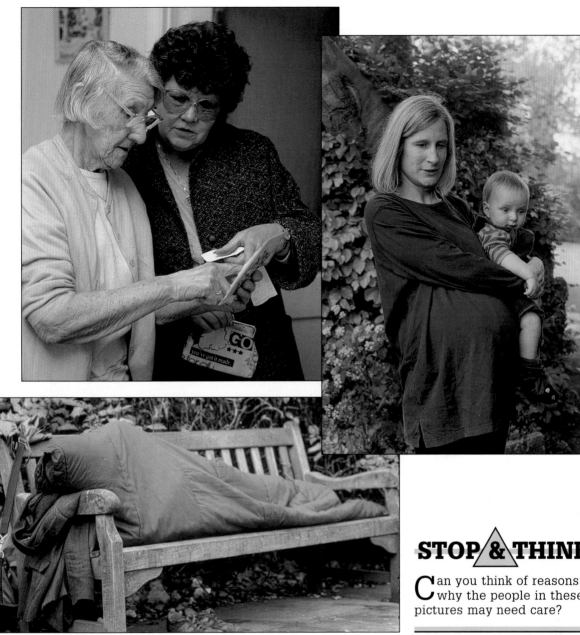

STOP & THINK

Can you think of reasons why the people in these pictures may need care?

People experience health, social and emotional difficulties when their needs are unmet. These difficulties may be related to their physical or mental health, their ability to learn skills or simply their ability to cope with everyday life. This is where care organisations and care workers can help.

Care organisations specialise in providing services that focus on the need for particular types of health, development or well-being. For example, maternity services specialise in providing services for women in the time leading up to, during and shortly after childbirth. This is because women have health care needs during pregnancy and childbirth that they often can't meet without help and support.

Quick Questions

1 What are the four types of basic need?

2 What can happen when a person has unmet needs?

3 What effects do you think childbirth might have on a woman's emotional needs?

Planning for different client groups

When care services are being developed, they are planned for groups of people who have the same type of problems or similar unmet needs. These groups of people are known as **client groups**. The client group targeted by maternity services, as we've just seen, are women from the time they are pregnant until shortly after childbirth. The client group targeted by most nursing and residential homes is older people (aged 65 years and over) who can't, or don't wish to, live in their own homes because they need care or support.

Care organisations in the United Kingdom provide health care, social care and education services that meet the physical, intellectual, social and emotional needs of major client groups. These client groups are:

- Babies and children (0–12)
- Adolescents (teenagers 13–16)
- Adults (16–65)
- Older people (65+)
- Disabled people (all ages)

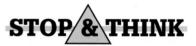

STOP & THINK

Can you think of any care services that are targeted at teenagers? What needs are these services aiming to meet?

As you can see, the client groups listed cover the whole of the human life span – from babies to very old people. Some people require care throughout their life, while others only use care services occasionally. The way that people use care services depends on a number of factors. One of these is the type of problem that they experience; another is the person's age and stage of development.

People at the same stage in life – childhood, adolescence or old age, for example – tend to have similar basic and developmental needs. Care organisations recognise this and target services at the unmet needs and the resulting health, social or developmental problems that members of a client group share.

CASE STUDY

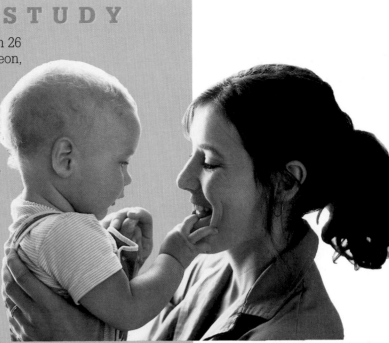

'My name is Nadine Burton. I'm 26 years old and have one child, Leon, who is now 9 months old. I've used care services quite a lot recently, mainly because of stress, and for Leon. I saw my GP [family doctor] when I felt under pressure and I wasn't sleeping well. I thought that he could give me something to help me sleep. Leon was waking up in the night and I had to get up to feed him all the time. I was tired all day and I wasn't coping very well. My neighbours then started complaining about Leon's crying. It made me feel depressed. The GP got me some help from social services.
They arranged for me to go to a mother and baby group. I now get to meet other new mums and we chat. I find it helps me to relax a bit. The GP also arranged for the Health Visitor to keep coming to see me. She gives me advice about feeding and caring for Leon and she's friendly. Things are getting easier now. Well, the neighbours have stopped complaining, anyway!'

- Which client group is Nadine a member of now?
- Which client group is Leon a member of?
- Give two reasons why Nadine needed help from care services.
- Explain how the care and support provided to Nadine help to meet her social and emotional needs.

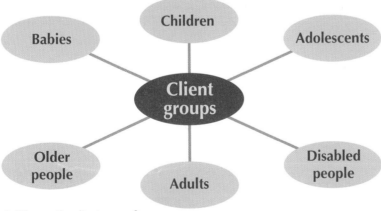

▲ Who are the client groups?

Quick Questions

1 What is a client group?
2 Why are care services planned for client groups?
3 Which client group do most nursing homes target their services at?

Babies

A newborn baby is unable to meet his or her own basic needs. Babies are dependent on others, usually their parents, to provide them with the things they need for growth and development. Growth involves the baby getting heavier and taller. Development involves improvement in the baby's skills.

For example, a baby will usually develop the ability to sit up and crawl before their first birthday. Examples of the things that babies and infants need to grow and develop in a healthy way include:

- food, clothing and warm shelter
- activity and sleep
- love and a sense of safety
- protection from illness and injury
- a carer they feel secure with and can trust
- praise and understanding to develop self-confidence
- stimulation to help them learn physical skills, language and social skills.

If you look at the list again, you'll see that a baby would be unable to meet their own need for any of the things listed. This is why babies and young children require so much care from others. To be healthy and to develop normally, babies require care from their parents and from care professionals.

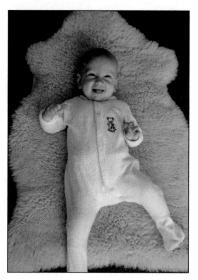

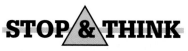
▲ What types of care might a baby need?

STOP & THINK

Can you think of two types of care worker who might provide some of the care a baby needs?

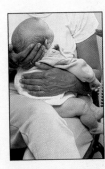

Baby's first year

Monday (age 4 weeks and 2 days) Danny can hold his head up on his own for a little while. He's still waking for lots of feeds in the night!

Wednesday (age 12 weeks) Rachel was pleased when Danny was able to hold the white rabbit she'd given him by himself. He still loves his food and giggles when he's bathed. Loves his cuddles, especially at bedtime!

Monday (age 6 months and 2 weeks) Danny turns his head very quickly to look at whoever's speaking. I don't think there's anything wrong with his hearing! He gets very excited when he hears Tom or Rachel.

He's started to get a bit fretful when anyone new visits us.

Friday (age 8 months and 3 weeks). Can sit up on his own. Doesn't go all floppy and keel over anymore! Pulls himself up on the furniture. Tom thinks he might walk soon.

Plays peek-a-boo with Rachel and calls her 'Rara'.

Sunday (age 1 year!) Took his first steps at his birthday party! Everyone was so excited. Gave Rachel a sloppy kiss when she hugged him. He thinks he's so clever! Wants to feed himself, but gets most of it in his hair or on the dog or anywhere but in his mouth. Does better with finger food and can use his cup OK.

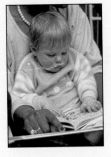

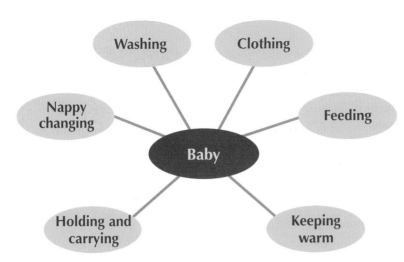

▲ The types of physical care that a baby needs

CASE STUDY

Luke is 2 months old. He had a normal birth. After a range of checks by the midwife and doctor at the hospital, his parents took him home the day after his birth. As a young baby, Luke is totally dependent on others for basic care and protection from harm. Luke's mother breast-feeds him several times during the day and night. She and his father take it in turns to change his nappy, wash him and comfort him when he starts crying. Luke's parents have to make sure that he is fed properly, that he is kept warm but that he doesn't get too hot and that he is kept clean and comfortable. Luke won't be able to meet these needs on his own until he is several years older.

- List any other basic needs that Luke has which you think are not mentioned in the case study (hint: what else does he need to be a healthy baby?).

- Identify two things that Luke's mother or father do that meet his physical needs.

- What kind of care worker comes to visit a mother and baby at home shortly after the birth to check that the baby is healthy and growing well?

Quick Questions

1 Name two skills that babies develop before their first birthday.
2 Why do babies need a lot of care?

Children

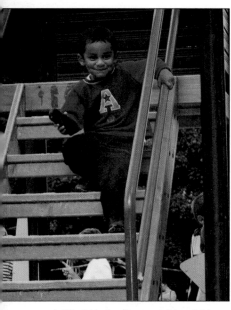

▲ What kinds of care might a child need?

From the age of three onwards children gradually become less dependent on their parents. They need less care from their parents as they learn how to meet some of their own basic needs. Even so, healthy children still need a balanced diet, good personal hygiene, exercise, rest, sleep, and opportunities to play and learn. In order to develop their skills and abilities children also need to:

- have friendships with other children
- have exercise and opportunities to take part in physical activities
- learn new skills and develop their basic knowledge (reading, writing, counting)
- have opportunities to learn how to behave with non-family members
- take responsibility for their behaviour and develop self-control
- develop self-care skills (washing, dressing, going to the toilet).

CASE STUDY

Anna is aged 3 years 6 months. She has recently begun attending a playgroup two mornings a week. Anna's mother helps to run the playgroup. She thinks that attending playgroup is good for Anna's development. When Anna is at the playgroup she meets and plays with up to ten other children. Anna enjoys playing with sand and water and now joins in games with other children. Her mother says that Anna has learnt how to make new friends and is much less shy than she was before she started going to playgroup.

- Why does Anna go to playgroup?
- What new skills or abilities might playgroup help Anna to develop?
- Explain how play might help Anna to develop intellectual skills.

STOP & THINK

Can you think of any other basic or specialist types of care a child might need to be healthy and happy?

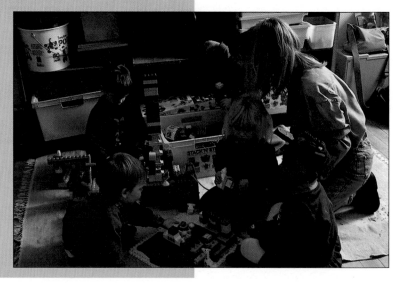

There are many care services for children. **Early years services** concentrate on helping young children to meet their developmental needs. They provide child care and education services for children under the age of eight. Play activities that help children to learn and develop their physical, intellectual and social skills are a common part of all early years services.

Local areas throughout the United Kingdom also have child health services that are designed to meet a range of health care needs. For example, a baby or child may require emergency health care services if they have an accident or develop a life-threatening illness or disease. However, this is unusual. On the other hand, as a routine precaution most children receive immunisations to protect them against childhood illnesses such as chicken pox, measles and mumps.

CASE STUDY

Last Christmas Ashok, aged 10, was admitted to a children's hospital when he fell over on his new roller blades. Ashok broke his ankle and banged his head hard against the pavement. He stayed in the children's hospital for three days while tests were done and his ankle was put in plaster. Ashok felt frightened and lonely in hospital and was glad to go home after his short stay.

- What care needs did Ashok have as a result of his accident?
- What effect did being in hospital have on Ashok's emotional well-being?
- List as many childhood illnesses as you can. Try to identify the types of care or treatment that are provided to deal with them.

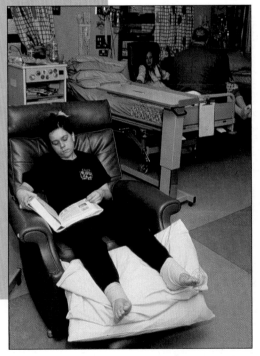

Social care needs of babies and children

Social care is a general term used to describe the support and non-medical care services provided for people who have personal, emotional or financial problems. Social care covers a broad range of care services, including foster care. **Foster care** is available to children and young people unable to live at home with their parents. Foster care placements are usually temporary. The child or young person lives with approved foster carers, who often have children of their own, until they are able to return home.

Quick Questions

1 What services do early years organisations provide for children?

2 Why do children have immunisations?

3 What does foster care involve?

Adolescents

What is an adolescent? You are, probably! An adolescent is a young person who is in the life stage between childhood and adulthood. A more common term for a person in this life stage is 'teenager'.

Adolescents are a distinct client group because they have care needs that are different from those of children and adults. During adolescence young people go through puberty. This involves major physical growth and development (see page 172 and 174) but doesn't normally involve teenagers experiencing major health problems. However, some teenagers do develop additional health needs that require specialist care and treatment. For example, teenage girls may require health care services for problems related to menstruation and many adolescents seek help for skin problems, such as acne, that often occur during puberty.

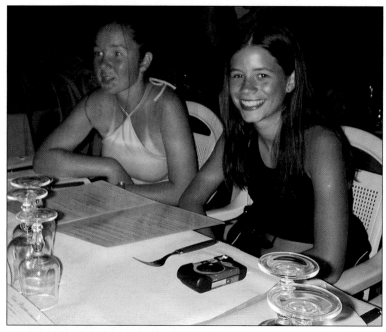

▲ Why might an adolescent need care?

During adolescence young people often require support to help them with their social and emotional development. For example, young people may require:

■ supportive relationships with parents and other adults

■ experiences that build up their confidence and self-esteem

■ opportunities to express their opinions and explore their own feelings

■ love and a sense of security

■ the chance to make personal decisions about their future

- opportunities to develop knowledge and skills useful for adult life and work
- opportunities to socialise and develop and express their sense of personal identity
- advice and guidance about relationships, sex and sexuality.

Young people sometimes need somebody outside their family to talk to about their relationships and feelings. Social care services, provided by specialist counsellors and youth workers, are available in some local areas to help meet the social and emotional needs that some adolescents have.

There aren't as many specialist care services for adolescents as there are for either babies and children or the adult client group. In some areas, adolescents are grouped together with all children under 16 years of age into a general 'children and young people' client group. This is often because there isn't enough money to provide separate services for adolescents, not because they have the same care needs as children.

CASE STUDY

Gina is 15 years old. She says she can't wait to leave school and get a job. Gina currently has a difficult relationship with her parents. She complains that they treat her like a child and are too strict with her. Gina believes that she is mature enough to make decisions for herself. Gina's parents complain that she has become 'very difficult' and that she no longer listens to what they tell her. They insist that she doesn't go out after school during the week and won't let her stay at friends' houses at the weekend. Gina feels too angry with her parents to talk to them about any of these things at the moment.

- Who could help Gina to express how she feels?
- What kind of physical care needs do adolescents like Gina have?
- Why do you think parents have difficult relationships with their children during adolescence?

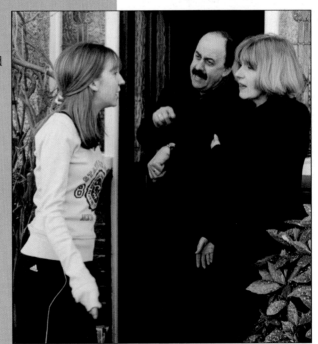

Quick Questions

1 What is puberty?
2 Why should adolescents receive different care services than children do?

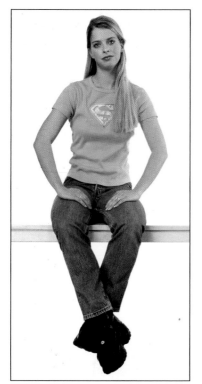

▲ What types of care might an adult need?

Adults

When is a person an adult rather than an adolescent? Is it when they reach their sixteenth birthday and are legally allowed to get married, leave school and begin full-time work? Or is it when they're 18 and they get the right to vote, have a credit card and buy alcohol? There is no precise answer, but care organisations usually include everyone between the ages of 16 and 65 years of age in their adult client group.

Care services for the adult client group have to cover a very wide range of health and social care needs. Adulthood is the longest life stage – there are 49 years between a person's sixteenth and their sixty-fifth birthdays – and a lot of things can happen that affect health and well-being during this period of life.

Adulthood is a life stage where people are usually more able to meet their own physical, intellectual, social and emotional needs independently. Adults are generally able to make their own decisions and take control of their own lives. But there are always situations in which people need help in meeting their needs or where they are unable to take control of their own life properly.

Self-reported health problems by gender and age

United Kingdom	Percentages				All aged 16 and over
	16–44	45–64	65–74	75+	
Males					
Pain or discomfort	18	39	52	56	32
Mobility	6	22	36	50	18
Anxiety or depression	12	19	20	19	15
Problems performing usual activities	5	16	21	27	12
Problems with self care	1	6	8	14	5
Females					
Pain or discomfort	20	40	51	65	34
Mobility	6	21	37	60	19
Anxiety or depression	18	24	25	30	22
Problems performing usual activities	7	17	23	40	15
Problems with self care	2	5	9	21	6

Source: *Social Trends 30*, © 2000 HMSO

OVER TO YOU

1. What percentage of men aged 16-44 reported that they had pain or discomfort?

2. Is the percentage of women in the same age group higher or lower?

3. What reasons could there be for this difference?

4. Overall, are men or women most likely to report having health problems?

5. How does a person's age seem to affect the likelihood of them reporting health problems?

Adults can have unexpected accidents or suffer illnesses and diseases that require specialist medical help and care. Some health problems, such as broken bones, can be treated and cured quickly. Other people have long-term, or chronic, health problems, for example heart disease or HIV infection, and need to use care services throughout their adult life. The same is also true of social care services. Some people may need help and support for a short period, such as when a child needs foster care, while other people need continuing support to help them cope with the stresses and difficulties in their lives.

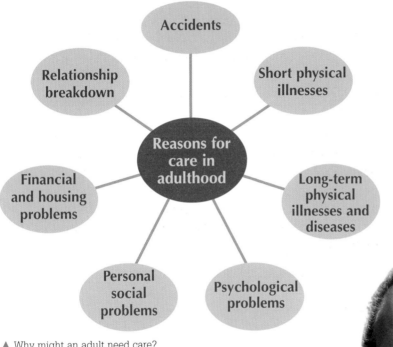

▲ Why might an adult need care?

CASE STUDY

Jimmy Davis is 49 years of age. He was made redundant nine months ago. He has applied for over a hundred jobs since then but still hasn't been able to get work. Jimmy has recently started to feel depressed, thinking that he will never get another job and that he is 'no good' because he can't find work. Jimmy's wife has started to worry about the way he is feeling and has suggested that he should go to see his GP to talk about it. Jimmy say's he'd be too embarrassed to talk about 'being a failure'.

- What kinds of health problems does Jimmy have at the moment?
- How do you think Jimmy could be helped to overcome his current health problems?
- List some of the health care services that an adult could use to look after and protect their health in a planned way.

Quick Questions

1 What is a chronic health problem?

2 At which age range are adult care services aimed?

Older people

'Older people' is the term used to describe the group of adults who are 65 years of age and over. It is seen as a more positive term than 'pensioner', 'old person' or 'the elderly'.

Older people are a major client group for care services. According to government statistics, the size of this client group is growing fast.

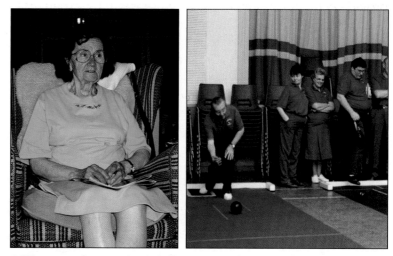

▲ What types of care might an older person need?

Population by gender and age in the UK

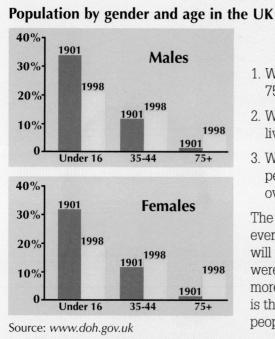

Source: *www.doh.gov.uk*

OVER TO YOU

1. What percentage of the female population was 75 or over in 1901?

2. Why do you think that so many more women lived to be 75 years or older in 1998 than in 1901?

3. What factors might explain the difference in the percentages of men and women living to 75 and over in 1998?

The statistics suggest that we're more likely than ever to survive into old age. For many people this will mean living into very old age. In 1951 there were less than 300 people aged 100 years old or more. By 1991 this had increased to 5,500 people. It is thought that there are likely to be over 40,000 people living to this age by 2036!

Every adult experiences the **ageing process**. This is a gradual process that involves changes to our bodies and our minds. The ageing process tends to reduce a person's physical ability and sometimes has an effect on intellectual (mental) ability. Our bodies aren't as strong and don't work as well in old age as they did during adolescence or early adulthood (see page 178 for more on this). Some older people require help and support to meet their basic needs as a result of the physical or mental problems that they experience during old age. However, it isn't true that all older people are frail and unwell.

Care organisations provide a wide range of services for older people. These aim to meet the basic and additional needs of older people. For example, specialist health care services provide care and treatment for older people who experience health care problems such as arthritis and heart disease. Older people are more likely to have these health problems than younger adults. Some older people also have unmet emotional needs because their partners and friends have died and they have difficulty in getting out and meeting other people. The sense of loss and isolation that some older people experience can result in them feeling depressed and lonely.

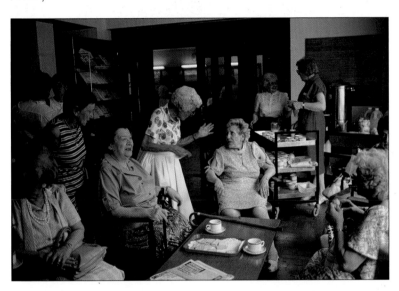

◄ Social events, such as coffee mornings and lunch clubs, can help to reduce the feelings of loneliness and isolation that some older people feel

Quick Questions

1 What is the ageing process?
2 Why do some older people require help from care services?

CASE STUDY

Mrs Jean Baker is 78 years of age. Until a year ago she spent most of her time looking after her house and her husband Peter, aged 80. Peter Baker had a severe heart attack a year ago and has been in hospital ever since. Mrs Baker tries to visit him whenever she can but is finding life on her own very difficult. She feels that she needs help to cope with her housework and general chores such as shopping. Mrs Baker has also been feeling unwell recently and has been lonely since her husband was admitted to hospital.

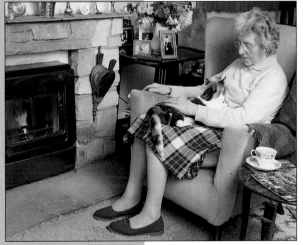

- What do you think Mrs Baker's care needs are?

- How could Mrs Baker be given more emotional support?

- Name two types of care service which are provided to meet the needs of older people.

Disabled people

The term 'disabled person' is used by care organisations to describe anyone who has a form of physical, sensory or intellectual impairment that causes them to have additional care needs beyond those of a non-disabled person of the same age. For example, someone who loses their sight continues to have the usual need for basic health care but may have an additional need for help and support to cope with other aspects of their daily life.

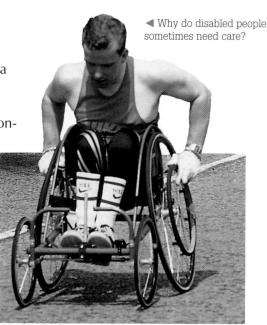

◄ Why do disabled people sometimes need care?

Disabled people have a wide variety of additional needs. Some disabled people require a lot of medical and health care because of their impairment or medical condition. Other disabled people require very little help from care services. A disabled person's need for care depends on their individual circumstances.

How can impairment affect people?

A person with a **sensory impairment** may have problems with their eyes (visual impairment) or their ears (hearing impairment). This type of impairment can affect a child's development unless the child receives specialist care services. For example, children who are unable to see or hear well may have development problems and their impairment may affect their learning unless specialist education is provided.

Physical impairment may affect people in many different ways. For example, problems such as spinal injury may cause someone to be paralysed from the waist or neck down. A disorder such as spina bifida affects how someone grows and develops, whereas a disorder such as cystic fibrosis affects the ways in which the body works. Some physical impairments shorten life, whereas others don't but may result in the person requiring care throughout a longer life span. Without appropriate care, support and treatment many physically disabled people would not be able to meet their own needs and would have poor quality of life.

Care organisations use the term **learning disability** to refer to the problems experienced by people who have an intellectual impairment. Learning difficulty services are provided for people of all ages who have limited ability to think and learn new things and, because of this, are unable

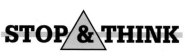

STOP & THINK

What kinds of additional help or care do you think a person might need if they lost their eyesight?

to take control of their own lives or live independently. For example, people who have Down's Syndrome have a learning disability for which specialist education and social care services are provided.

Care services for disabled people

Disabled people are a large client group for whom a range of specialist health, social care and early years services are provided. Care services for disabled people cover all age ranges, from babies to older people. Care organisations try to suit the services they provide both to the age of the disabled person as well as to their impairment. In many local areas, services for disabled people are organised into services for disabled children, services for disabled adults and services for disabled older people to ensure that individual needs can be properly met.

CASE STUDY

Richard is 32 years of age and was born with Down's Syndrome. He lives at home with his parents and attends a day centre where he has made some friends. Richard has learnt to wash, dress and feed himself but requires help and support to adapt to new people and changes in his routine. Richard's parents and carers say that he is not yet able to make decisions for himself or live independently. Even so, Richard says that he'd like to be a bus driver and get married one day.

- What kinds of care needs do you think Richard has at the moment?

- Explain how going to the day centre could help to meet Richard's needs.

- How do you think Richard could be helped to become more independent?

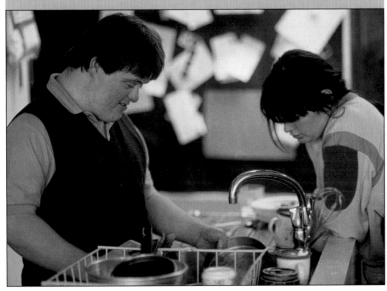

Quick Questions

1 What is a sensory impairment?
2 Name one cause of physical impairment.
3 Why is it incorrect to assume that all disabled people need a lot of care?

Build your learning

LEARNING POINTS

The following are the main points that you should have learnt from the previous 16 pages.

- People need care in all stages of life.

- The sort of care that people require depends on their needs and problems.

- Care services are provided to meet the particular needs of client groups (babies, children and adults, for example) who are in the same life stage and have similar needs and problems.

- Care services are planned to meet the needs of members of client groups who live in the same local area.

REVISION QUESTIONS

If you're confident that you understand the learning points and the key terms, try answering the revision questions below:

1 Identify the five major client groups for which care services are provided.

2 Describe the basic care needs of a baby.

3 Explain how local care services are planned.

The key question you should now be able to answer if you've understood the previous section is:

4 'Who needs care and why?'

KEY TERMS

You should know what the following terms mean:
- Basic needs (page 10)
- Unmet needs (page 10)
- Client groups (page 12)
- Early years service (page 17)
- Social care (page 17)
- Foster care (page 17)
- Puberty (page 18)
- The ageing process (page 22)
- Sensory impairment (page 24)
- Physical impairment (page 24)
- Learning disability (page 24)

If you're not sure or want to check your understanding, turn to the page number listed in the brackets.

INVESTIGATION IDEAS

1 Find out about the types of care services that exist in your local area. Produce a map or directory of all the local care services provided for the different client groups in your area. You may want to do this as part of a group, with each person concentrating on a different client group.

2 Obtain information about your local population by contacting your local authority or health authority.

Try to obtain a copy of the plans that they've made for providing care services to the local community over the next few years. You might get this information by writing to them and asking for a copy of the local community care plan or health services plan. Alternatively, you could search for the information on their website and look for articles about it in your local newspapers.

Developing local care services

In the previous pages we looked at client groups and the general reasons why care services are provided for each group. We said that care services for each client group aim to help people with health or social problems or with their growth and development. But who decides which services should be provided in the first place? Why are some care services available in your local area but not others?

Think about the types of care services that exist in your area. There are probably quite a few local family doctors, dentists and perhaps opticians. You will also have a local social services department that offers social work services. Do you know why you've got these services and not others?

Care services are planned and provided to meet the needs of different client groups. To offer the services that are required by local people, care organisations need to know who lives in their area and what kinds of problems they have. For example, in order to provide maternity services, local health care organisations need to know how many women of childbearing age live in their area and how many children are likely to be born in a year. How can they get this information? One way is to carry out a survey of the local population. The survey will give care organisations information that helps them to predict the likely maternity care needs of local people. Care organisations also collect information about the people who use their services throughout the year. The statistics they produce help them to adjust their services as people's needs change and are also used to plan services for future years.

Local care organisations try to plan and develop services to meet local care needs. At the same time, they are required by government to provide services that are seen as priorities because they deal with national problems. For example, drug misuse services, services for homeless people and services that reduce child poverty. We will look at examples of these types of care services later in this unit.

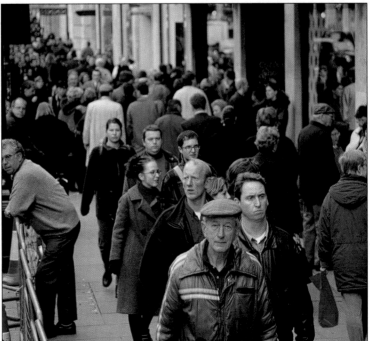

▼ Care services must be planned to meet the diverse needs of local people

The care system

You probably know of a number of different health, social care and early years services in your local area. There may be a hospital, a health centre, a family doctor (GP) service, a nursery or a residential home near to where you live, for example. You may have used some of these services yourself, or perhaps members of your family have used them.

Local care services such as those mentioned above are available from a range of different organisations and self-employed care workers. Care services provided by care organisations and by self-employed practitioners are known as formal services. However, when you think about providers of care, don't forget that family, friends and even neighbours may also be important providers of care for some people. Many people turn to their parents, partner or close friends first when they need basic care or support for a health or personal problem. The care that these people provide is called informal care. We need to include informal care when we look at the various types of care services that exist in the United Kingdom.

Taken together, all the care organisations, self-employed practitioners and informal carers who provide care throughout the United Kingdom make up what is called the care system. In the next section of this unit we take a closer look at the different types of organisations that exist within the care system, and at the ways they are organised.

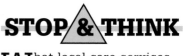

STOP & THINK

What local care services have you used recently?

Quick Questions

- Do self-employed care workers provide formal or informal care?
- Explain the difference between formal and informal care services.

The four care sectors

One way of making the care system easier to understand is to divide it up into four different parts or 'sectors'. These are known as the statutory, voluntary, private and informal care sectors.

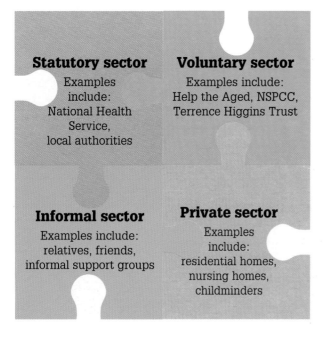

Statutory sector
Examples include:
National Health Service,
local authorities

Voluntary sector
Examples include:
Help the Aged, NSPCC,
Terrence Higgins Trust

Informal sector
Examples include:
relatives, friends,
informal support groups

Private sector
Examples include:
residential homes,
nursing homes,
childminders

The statutory care sector

The government is responsible for controlling and running the part of the care system known as the statutory sector. This care sector includes organisations such as the National Health Service (NHS) and local authorities (local councils). These organisations provide most health, social care and early years services throughout the United Kingdom. The government has a legal duty to provide some types of care services. The laws that set out these duties are called statutes. This is where the term statutory comes from. We will look at services provided by the statutory sector in more detail later in this unit (see pages 30–9).

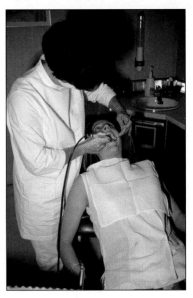

▲ Many dentists provide both statutory (NHS) and private dental services

The private sector

The private sector is made up of care businesses and individual self-employed practitioners, such as private nurseries, childminders and dentists for example. Private sector organisations and self-employed practitioners usually charge people a fee for the health, social care or early years services that they provide. Private sector care providers work to make a profit as well as to meet care needs.

The voluntary care sector

The voluntary care sector is made up of organisations that are not controlled by government. Voluntary organisations provide their care services because they see a need for them. They don't have a legal (or statutory) duty to do this but do so voluntarily. Scope is an example of a voluntary sector organisation that works with people who have learning disabilities. Voluntary organisations provide a large range of care services in the United Kingdom. They are independent from the government and non-profit making.

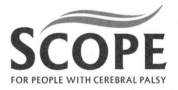

SCOPE
FOR PEOPLE WITH CEREBRAL PALSY

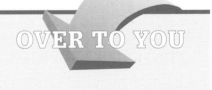

OVER TO YOU

Use the internet, your local library, your GP surgery, health centre or a telephone directory to identify private practitioners in your local area.

The informal sector

The informal sector consists of the very large number of unpaid informal carers who look after members of their own family, friends or neighbours who have care needs. Care providers in each of the four sectors make an important contribution to the overall delivery of care services in the United Kingdom. There are important differences in the type of service that practitioners and organisations in the different sectors offer. However, there are also many areas in which they work together (see page 46).

Quick Questions

1 What are the four different care sectors in the United Kingdom called?
2 Which sector covers the care given by relatives, friends and neighbours?

We learnt in the last section that the statutory sector provides care services funded (paid for) by government because the law requires them to. This hasn't always been the case. The statutory care system began only in 1948 when the government took on responsibility for providing care services and began to develop what became known as a welfare state. This was to be a system of free health, social care and education for all citizens of the United Kingdom.

Before this, health services were not available for everyone. Some voluntary services existed, but most people had to pay a doctor privately or join an insurance scheme if they wanted health care. This meant that most people didn't receive good health care services because they couldn't afford to pay.

The National Health Service (NHS) was launched in 1948 to tackle problems of ill-health and provide services for everyone in the United Kingdom. It has been the main provider of statutory health care services ever since. Local authorities (local councils) also have close links with the beginning of the welfare state in 1948. They have a long history of providing statutory social care and education services in local areas throughout the United Kingdom.

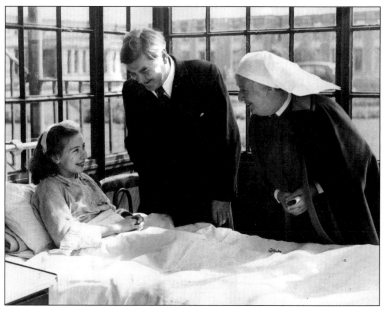

▲ The young girl in bed was the first ever NHS patient. She is pictured meeting Aneurin Bevan, the Minister of Health responsible for launching the NHS on 1 May 1948

Statutory health, social care and early years services today

The two care organisations that provide most statutory care services today are the National Health Service and local authorities. Local authorities provide social care, housing and education services for people of all ages in a defined local area. Examples of the statutory services they provide include emergency health care, schooling up to the age of 16 and housing for homeless people. The NHS and local authorities also purchase (buy) services for clients from voluntary and private sector organisations. Even though they are not providing these services directly, this allows them to fulfil their legal responsibilities to provide certain types of care.

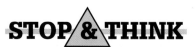

Do you think that health care should always be free or should people be charged for some types of services?

What part does the government play in the statutory care sector?

The government of the United Kingdom is made up of politicians who are members of the political party that has won the previous general election. Making sure that health care is provided is one of the main tasks of every government. The Department of Health is the part of government that is responsible for planning and managing statutory health and social care services. Government politicians and civil servants at the Department of Health make decisions about how statutory health care services should be organised and paid for throughout the country. The politician who has overall responsibility for this is called the Secretary of State for Health.

The government is the main provider of the money for statutory care services. This government money (also called 'funding') is used to employ thousands of people in a wide variety of care jobs, buy equipment and keep the statutory system running. The government funds most hospitals, social service departments and state schools in the United Kingdom.

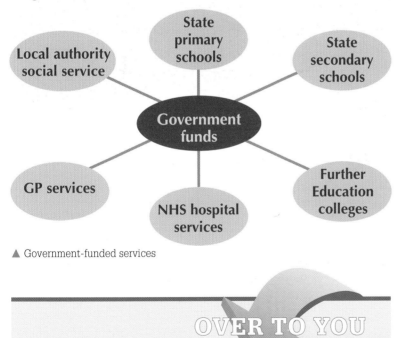

▲ Government-funded services

OVER TO YOU

You can find out more about the NHS and the welfare state by searching government and educational sites on the internet. Try these sites to get started:

- www.doh.gov.uk/
- www.nhs.uk/

Quick Questions

1 What does the term 'statutory' mean?

2 Explain why the statutory system was developed in 1948.

3 Which government department plans statutory health and social care services?

Health care

Most of us will have contact with the statutory health care services at some point in our lives, either for emergency care or more usually because we have a less severe illness and go to a GP (family doctor) for help. Statutory health care organisations provide medical assessment and treatment as well as specialist care services aimed at tackling illness and improving health. These services include nursing, occupational therapy and physiotherapy for people of all ages who have physical or psychological problems.

Statutory health care services are mainly provided by organisations that are a part of the National Health Service. All local areas throughout England and Wales have an NHS Trust organisation that has overall responsibility for statutory health care in the area. Local NHS Trust organisations provide hospital and community-based health care services for people of all ages.

Statutory health care organisations provide two main types of service:

- Primary health care services
- Secondary health care services

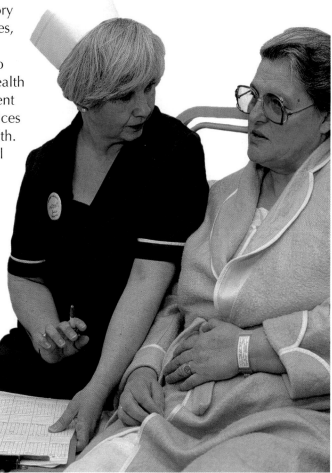

▲ Statutory health care organisations provide a range of nursing services

Primary health care services

Primary health care services include the basic, usually non-emergency types of health care. Most people use primary health care services when they first have worries about their health, when they have a minor illness or when they need to get their health checked. Some people need to use primary health care services regularly because they have a health problem or disability that requires continuing treatment or monitoring.

Primary health care services are provided in community settings, such as health centres, clinics and people's homes. Primary health care workers provide health care for all client groups in the local population. Primary health care services are delivered by a number of health care staff working together as a primary health care team (PHCT). A general practitioner (GP or family doctor) is often the leader or co-ordinator of the team. Other team members include practice nurses, district nurses, community psychiatric nurses and health visitors. Team members meet regularly to discuss clients and co-ordinate their work with them. This helps to ensure that patients receive the best possible treatment.

◀ Health centres provide many care services for the local community

Brentford Lodge

Hounslow Primary Care NHS Trust **NHS**
www.hounslowpct.nhs.uk

Brentford Health Centre

General Practitioners:

Dr Lane, Dr Jones, Dr Roy, Dr Gupta	020 8321 3844
Dr Yasin,	020 8321 3822
Dr Crowe, Dr Lawrence & Dr Baxter	020 8321 3838

Community Health Service Enquiries   Tel: 020 8321 3800

Counselling	Leg Ulcer Clinic
Podiatry	Macmillan & Marie Curie Nursing
District Nursing	School Nursing
Family Planning/Well Woman	Speech & Language Therapy
Health Visiting	Stoma & Continence Nursing
	Physiotherapy

As well as treating the health problems that people already have, primary health care workers also provide a range of check-ups, clinics and classes aimed at improving health and preventing illness. You may have seen these things publicised in leaflets or on posters at your own health centre. Common examples of health improvement services include weight-loss clinics, stopping smoking and stress-reduction classes.

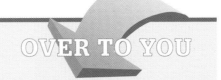

OVER TO YOU

Teenagers often feel that their health needs should be taken more seriously. Suggest two services that you think primary health care workers should offer to teenagers at your local health centre. Briefly explain your reasons.

Quick Questions

1 Name two types of health care service that are provided by statutory health care organisations.

2 What is a primary health care team?

3 List three things that primary health care workers offer to improve people's health and prevent illness.

Specialist health services

The specialist types of care and treatment provided in a hospital or a specialist clinic are known as secondary care. This type of care also includes some community health care services, such as district nursing services for people with long-term problems. Generally, community health care services are forms of care and treatment provided outside of hospital in a patient's own home or in a day centre, for example.

Hospital care services focus on specific, and often complex, health problems rather than on general and everyday problems. For example, large general hospitals usually have an accident and emergency department to deal with both life-threatening and minor injuries, a theatre or surgical department to deal with operations and a maternity unit to deal with childbirth. All these departments provide specialised health care services.

As well as providing complex care and treatment services, hospitals often have specialist services such as laboratories and radiography (X-ray) departments. These are used to diagnose (identify) health problems that GPs and other primary care workers are unable to identify because they don't have the specialist facilities or knowledge.

Most secondary hospital care is provided by NHS Trust hospitals. These are government-funded organisations that have a legal responsibility to provide health care services locally. There are a number of different kinds of hospital.

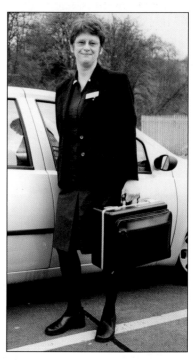

▲ Community nurses visit clients at home and in other non-hospital settings

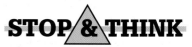

STOP & THINK

What kinds of events or situations can result in adults needing urgent care or treatment from secondary health care services?

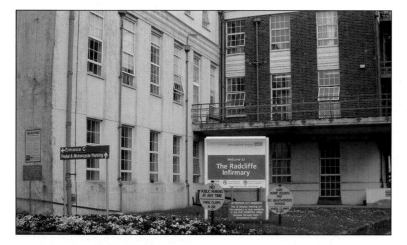

■ District General Hospitals provide a wide range of secondary health care services for the whole population of an area. For example, they provide services for seriously ill adults and for children who need an operation or treatment involving contact with specially trained doctors and nurses.

■ Local community hospitals usually provide a more limited range of treatments for a smaller number of people in an area. They often have facilities for people to be seen as outpatients and have far fewer beds than district general hospitals.

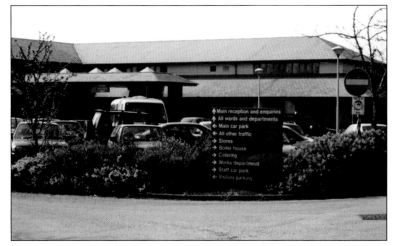

▲ Community hospitals provide non-specialist nursing and medical care locally

■ National Teaching Hospitals and Specialist Units provide highly specialised medical, surgical and psychiatric treatment for patients who come from all over the United Kingdom. Their expertise is available to both inpatients and outpatients. Examples of this kind of hospital are Great Ormond Street Hospital for Sick Children and the Royal Homeopathic Hospital (both in central London) and the Rampton High Security Hospital near Nottingham.

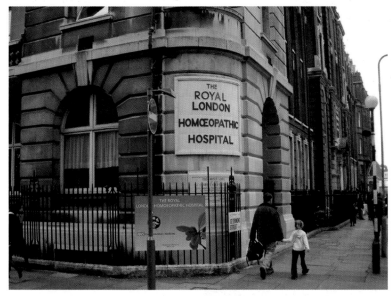

▲ Some hospitals, like this one, offer specialist treatment services to people from all over the United Kingdom

Quick Questions

1 Name three different local statutory health care organisations that provide secondary care services for babies, adolescents and older people.

2 What is community health care?

3 Which local organisations provide mental health care in your local area?

OVER TO YOU

Investigate the services offered by your nearest NHS Trust hospital. What kinds of specialist care and treatment are provided for children? Does the hospital specialise in any other kinds of health care service? Write a brief description summarising the health care services available at the hospital.

Social care

Social care services are forms of non-medical help and support that are provided for people who are vulnerable; either temporarily or over a long period of time. Such people require social care because they are unable to meet their personal and social needs independently.

The social services departments of local authorities have responsibility for statutory social care services. The purchasing section of a social services department buys care services for adult clients whose social care needs have been assessed. The services that are purchased are known as a care package.

The provider section of a social services department delivers some of the care services local people need, especially social work services. However, the purchasing section can also pay voluntary and private sector organisations to provide the care services that their adult clients need.

Local authorities also provide statutory social care services for children. The Children Act 1989 makes social services departments legally responsible for the welfare of children in need. For example, social services departments must provide child protection services, services for children under five and accommodation for children who are unable to live with their families.

What part does the government play in the statutory social care sector?

The Secretary of State for Health is the government minister (a politician) who has overall responsibility for making sure that statutory social care services are provided. The Department of Health, which includes the Social Services Inspectorate (SSI), is the part of government that plans and manages statutory social care services. The government provides the money (funding) needed to supply statutory social care services and employ all of the staff who deliver them. The SSI also provides guidance to Local Authorities about social care, and monitors and inspects the performance of social services departments.

STOP & THINK

Why do you think home help services are classified as social care rather than health care services?

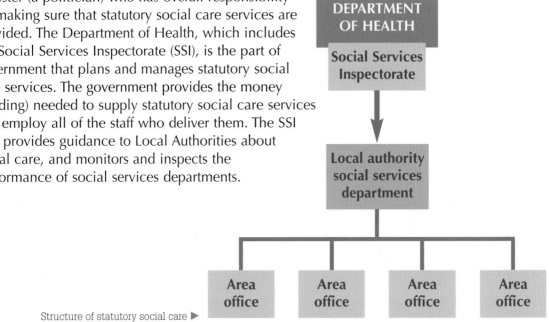

Structure of statutory social care ▶

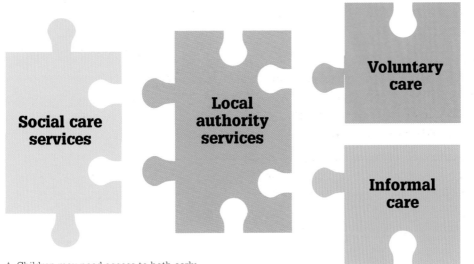

Social care services

Local authority services

Voluntary care

Informal care

▲ Children may need access to both early years services and social care services

CASE STUDY

When Sian was 10 years old her mother, a lone parent, was admitted to hospital with a serious illness. Sian, her mother and a social worker decided together that the best option was for Sian to live with foster carers. Sian lived with the Wilson family for three months until she returned to live at home with her mother. Sian said she missed her mum a lot at first and felt she didn't fit in but she did grow to like the Wilsons. She still gets a birthday card from them.

- Why did Sian need care at this point in her life?
- What kinds of care and support do you think a foster carer would provide for a child like Sian?
- When Sian was missing her mother, which of her needs were unmet?

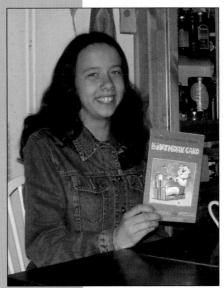

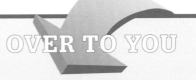

OVER TO YOU

Foster care is a form of social care that is provided for children and adolescents. You can find out more about what this involves at the Fostering Network site on the internet. The address is www.fostering-network.org.uk

Quick Questions

1 Give two reasons why people may need social care services.

2 Which organisation is responsible for providing statutory social care services in your local area?

3 Which government department is responsible for planning statutory social care services?

Early years

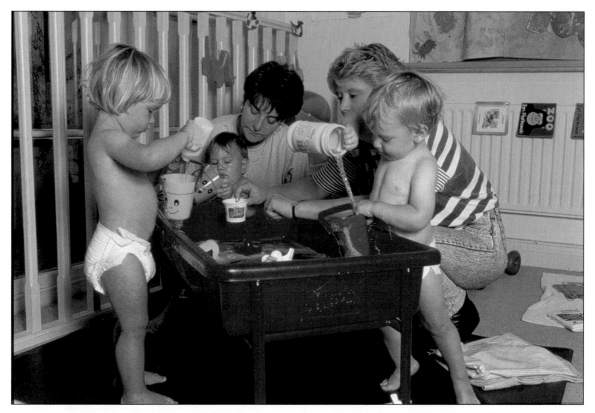

▲ Early years provision focuses on child care and early education

Early years organisations provide child care and development services for children under the age of eight. There are very few statutory child care services in the United Kingdom. This is because child care in the United Kingdom is generally seen as the responsibility of parents and other relatives of children. However, the government and local authority organisations are involved in providing some early years services.

Who provides local early years services?

Local authorities are responsible for purchasing (buying) early years care for children in need in their area. Early years care and education services are usually provided by the social services department and education department of a local authority.

Statutory early years services are only provided for families when a child is 'at risk' or where family pressures and problems can be reduced by child care support. Children with disabilities or those who have health or development problems are also eligible for these statutory services. Examples of early years services for children include playgroups, nurseries, childminders and family centres.

Children and families who use these services must have unmet care and development needs that have been identified by a social worker or other early years professional.

The main legal duties that local authorities have for early years services are contained in the Children Act 1989. This law requires that all people providing a childminder service, and the premises in which they care for the children, must be assessed and registered by their local authority. It is the legal responsibility of the social services department to carry out childminder assessments and to keep a register of approved childminders.

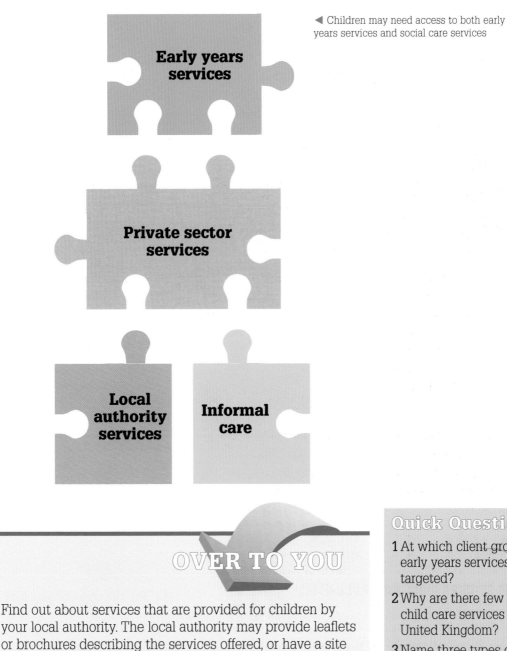

◀ Children may need access to both early years services and social care services

Early years services

Private sector services

Local authority services

Informal care

OVER TO YOU

Find out about services that are provided for children by your local authority. The local authority may provide leaflets or brochures describing the services offered, or have a site on the internet that you can look at.

Quick Questions

1 At which client group are early years services targeted?

2 Why are there few statutory child care services in the United Kingdom?

3 Name three types of early years service.

The care system in the United Kingdom includes a large voluntary sector. Voluntary sector care organisations are independent of government. The sector is called voluntary because many of the organisations have workers who are unpaid volunteers and also because the organisations provide their services voluntarily. Unlike statutory (government) organisations, they are not under a legal duty to do so.

Origins of the voluntary care sector

The voluntary care sector began in the nineteenth century when there were very few care services for ordinary people. At the time, most care services had to be paid for and were too expensive for all but the rich. Charities and voluntary organisations grew out of the campaigns and donations of a few rich philanthropists. These were wealthy individuals, such as Joseph Rowntree, who wanted to help their local communities and reduce the poverty and suffering they saw around them.

The voluntary sector now includes large organisations that work throughout the United Kingdom, as well as very small groups that work for a cause in their local area. National voluntary organisations include MENCAP, which campaigns for people with learning difficulties, Help the Aged, which works on behalf of older people, and the National Society for the Prevention of Cruelty to Children (NSPCC). Large voluntary organisations like these tend to have local branches and a national head office that co-ordinates the organisation's work around the country.

Large voluntary organisations provide a range of services. These include advice; telephone helplines; information about the issues affecting the people they work for and, in some cases, direct care services including housing, care homes and employment for vulnerable people.

▲ Joseph Rowntree was a wealthy man who gave money to help the poor in the nineteenth century

NSPCC

Cruelty to children must stop. FULL STOP.

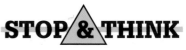

Barnardo's

GIVING CHILDREN BACK THEIR FUTURE

STOP & THINK

What kind of care-related work would you volunteer to do?

The very many small voluntary groups that exist in the United Kingdom are usually concerned with a highly specific or local issue, or provide a service to meet a particular local need. An example might be a support group for single parents or a local playgroup that aims to meet the needs of a group of children with autism.

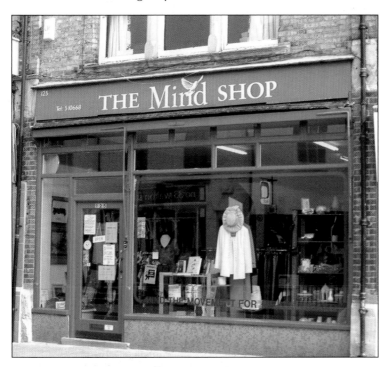

◄ MIND is a charity working on behalf of people with mental health problems

Most voluntary sector organisations are registered charities. This means that they obtain money to finance their services by fundraising for voluntary donations. Voluntary organisations sometimes also receive government grants, or small payments from the people they help, but they put their income back into running their services and don't try to make a profit. Voluntary organisations recruit many unpaid volunteers who provide their time and skills for free, but they also employ some care workers, managers and administrative staff as paid employees.

▼ A registered charity

Dogs for the Disabled

Reg. Charity No. 700454

How do we train our dogs

For the first year of their life, our puppies are homed with volunteers.

Here they learn basic social skills and commands and get to try out different situations that they may encounter during their working life, going to the shops or travelling on the bus.

After a lifetime's work, our dogs have earned a well-deserved retirement. Many stay on as a pet dog when a new working dog comes along, although some of them enjoy the work so much they carry on helping with their favourite task!

Jamie & Kandy

"Kandy helps me with so many tasks, but as well as assisting me everyday, she is like a close friend. She never grumbles or complains. Even better, I have made lots of new friends since getting Kandy, because just having a dog opens up new conversations. She has helped me increase my independence – and we have so much fun together"
Jamie, Client.

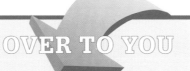

OVER TO YOU

Find out about the voluntary organisations that provide services for people in your local area. Try to identify at least one organisation that works on behalf of children, one for disabled people and one for older people.

Quick Questions

1 What is a philanthropist?

2 Explain why voluntary organisations developed in the late nineteenth century.

3 Do voluntary groups only employ volunteers?

The private care sector includes a range of private businesses and self-employed care workers. Private sector care businesses and **private practitioners** charge their clients fees in order to run their services and make a profit.

The private sector offers fewer services and has fewer organisations and service users than either the statutory or voluntary sectors. Within the private sector there are many more health care and early years organisations than social care organisations. Many of the services that are provided in the private sector cannot be obtained in the statutory system and are specialist, non-emergency services.

Health care

Private sector health care organisations include a number of large care businesses, such as BUPA and Nuffield Hospitals. These organisations provide complex health care services, including surgery, in their own private hospitals. It is also possible to pay for care as a private patient in a ward or unit of a National Health Service hospital. As well as hospitals and other direct care services, the private sector also includes a large number of employment agencies. These agencies specialise in recruiting and providing health care staff to other statutory, voluntary and private care organisations.

Private sector health care clients use health insurance to pay the costs of their care or pay the costs directly from their own funds.

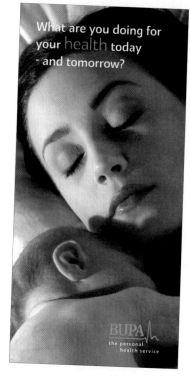

What are you doing for your health today - and tomorrow?

BUPA
the personal health service

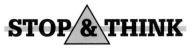

STOP & THINK

Why do you think some people choose to pay for private health care services?

Social care

There are very few social care organisations in the private sector. Those that do exist tend to provide specialised residential care services for older people or disabled people, or offer **domiciliary** (home) **care** services. People who use private sector social care services either have to pay for the cost of the services themselves or, if they meet the eligibility criteria, they may have their fees paid by their local authority social services department.

Early years services

Early years services in the private sector include nursery schools, playgroups, crèches and childminding services. These organisations provide child care and early education services to young children who have needs that are not met by the limited range of statutory sector services. As a child's parents must be able to afford to pay the fees, private sector child care services are not available to everyone who might need or benefit from them.

Self-employed carers and private practitioners

Health care workers such as dentists, physiotherapists and opticians, and social care workers such as counsellors and psychotherapists, sometimes offer their services through a private practice. This means that they are self-employed.

Sometimes they provide clients with an alternative service to those freely available from local statutory or voluntary sector organisations. In other circumstances they offer specialist services that are not available in the statutory or voluntary sector. An example might be osteopathy or acupuncture.

Some carers also work in their own homes on a self-employed basis. For example, registered childminders are the largest group of self-employed carers working in this way. Like all self-employed carers, they charge the people who use their services a fee for their time and expertise.

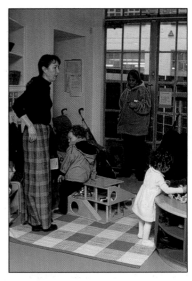

▲ Most early years care is provided by the private sector

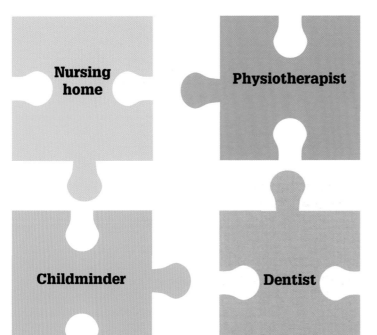

▲ Pieces in the private care jigsaw

Nursing home

Physiotherapist

Childminder

Dentist

Quick Questions

1 Name two specialist care services that are available in the private health care sector.

2 Name two ways that a person could pay for private health or social care.

3 Explain what domiciliary care involves.

OVER TO YOU

Find out about the range of private care services available to people in your local area. Try to identify at least one service for children, adults and older people.

INFORMAL CARE SERVICES

Many people who need care and support are not catered for in the formal care system. Instead, care and support are provided by unpaid, and often untrained, people such as relatives, friends and neighbours. This type of care is known as informal care.

Most of the health and social care for sick and vulnerable people in the United Kingdom is provided by people who look after relatives or friends. The vast majority of child care for children under five is also provided in this way. Children, older people and those with long-term care needs receive most informal care services. It's very common for people to provide care for their elderly relatives and children at home.

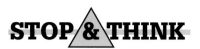

STOP & THINK

Do you provide informal care for anyone at present? How might this change later in your life?

CASE STUDY

Mrs Bell is 79 years old and lives alone. She has some memory impairment and forgets what time of the day it is, whether she has eaten, and also the names of all but her closest relatives and her neighbour, Mrs Scott. Mrs Bell is unable to walk any distance due to her arthritis, very rarely goes out alone, and is frightened to use her bath as she has difficulty getting in and out.

- What forms of informal care would Mrs Bell benefit from?

- Who might be able to provide each form of informal care for Mrs Bell?

- If you were a relative or neighbour of Mrs Bell's, how would you feel about giving up some of your time to offer Mrs Bell informal care and support?

Informal support groups

Support groups are another important way in which informal care is provided in the United Kingdom. There are many thousands of local, informal support groups operating throughout the United Kingdom at the present time. They are set up and run by carers and people who have special health and social care needs. For example, older people who care for a partner who has become frail or unwell may join together to form a local support group so that they can meet and gain support from each other. The groups may be small and short term, or may have become well established and provide regular, continuing support to an individual or a group of clients.

The purpose of informal support groups is to provide practical and emotional support to informal carers and the people they care for. An informal support group may consist of neighbours who share child care arrangements, people in a local area who all look after a relative alone at home, or a group of people who have got together to raise money to help an individual to finance his or her medical or social care needs.

Quick Questions

1 Name three groups of people who provide informal care services.
2 Which client groups are most likely to receive informal care?
3 Explain the main purpose of informal support groups.

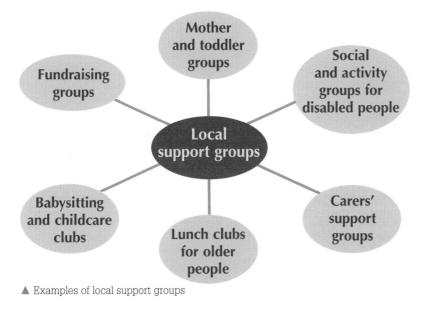

▲ Examples of local support groups

What kinds of informal support groups exist in your local area? Find out by looking for posters and leaflets in places like the local library, the sports centre, church halls, mosques or synagogues and in local day centres.

OVER TO YOU

Working together

So far we've looked at how the care system in the United Kingdom is organised into four different sectors. We've also considered the types of care services that are provided by local care organisations. This may have given you the impression that the different care sectors work separately from each other. While this may have been the case in the past, lots of effort is now being put into getting care organisations to work together.

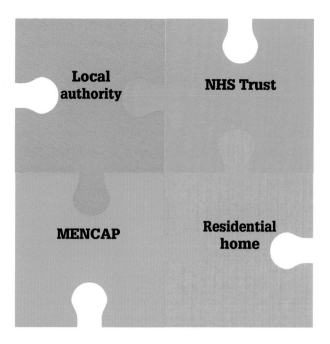

▲ Different types of organisations cooperate to provide care

Health authorities, NHS Trusts and local authority social services departments are now working together to 'modernise' local care services. In some areas this involves developing new Health and Social Care Trust organisations. The aim of this joint working between different types of care organisation is to reduce the costs of providing care and improve the efficiency and effectiveness of local care services. Better quality care services should result from new initiatives, such as health action zones and local health improvement programmes.

It is likely that organisations from different care sectors are working together to provide services for clients in your local area. For example, voluntary sector organisations such as MENCAP and SCOPE often work with statutory health organisations and local authority social services departments to provide care services for people with learning disabilities.

Increasingly, statutory sector health and social care organisations are also working with private sector organisations to ensure that people get the care they need. For example, many local authority social services departments now purchase (buy) care for older people in private sector nursing and residential homes. NHS Trusts who are unable to provide operations and other treatment for people on their waiting lists are also now buying this care and treatment for their patients from the private sector. It is likely that organisations in different care sectors will develop closer links and work together even more in the future.

Build Your Learning

LEARNING POINTS

The following are the main points that you should have learnt from the previous 20 pages.

- A wide range of care services is provided in the United Kingdom by organisations, private practitioners and informal carers

- The National Health Service (NHS) and local authority social services departments are the main statutory (state) sector care providers.

- Health care organisations provide primary and secondary care services in community and hospital settings.

- Social care organisations help people with a wide range of social, financial and emotional problems.

- Care organisations and private practitioners from all care sectors are increasingly working together both to help people with care needs and to support their informal carers.

REVISION QUESTIONS

If you're confident that you understand the learning points and the key terms, try answering the revision questions below:

1 Identify the four main care sectors.

2 Describe the reasons why voluntary sector care organisations developed in the United Kingdom.

3 Explain the difference between:
a) primary and secondary health care
b) a district general and a local community hospital
c) a voluntary sector and a private sector organisation.

The key question you should now be able to answer if you've understood the previous section is:

4 'What types of care services are provided to meet client group needs?'

KEY TERMS

You should know what the following terms mean:
- Formal services (page 28)
- Informal care (page 28)
- The care system (page 28)
- Statutory sector (page 29)
- National Health Service (page 29)
- Voluntary care sector (page 29)
- Private sector (page 29)
- Informal sector (page 29)
- Local authorities (page 30)
- Department of Health (page 31)
- NHS Trust (page 32)
- Primary health care (page 32)
- Secondary care (page 34)
- Community health care (page 34)
- Social care (page 36)
- Care package (page 36)
- Early years care (page 38)
- Philanthropists (page 40)
- Private practitioners (page 42)
- Domiciliary care (page 42)

If you're not sure or want to check your understanding, turn to the page number listed in the brackets.

INVESTIGATION IDEAS

1 Produce a list or map of local care organisations. Label the organisations on the list or map according to the care sector that they are part of and whether they are health, social care or early years organisations.

2 Research two local care organisations in detail. You may be able to obtain information by visiting them, by writing to them or, if they have one, by searching their website. Produce a profile of the organisations outlining:
a) the main services they offer
b) which sector each organisation belongs to
c) ways of obtaining their services
d) their sources of funding.

Ways of obtaining care services

How can people obtain the care services they need? While reading through this unit you may have realised that there are different ways of obtaining care services. As well as looking at the different ways people can obtain the care services they need, we are also going to look at the reasons why people sometimes don't get the services they require.

Referrals

The process of applying for, or requesting, a care service is known as referral. There are three main types of referral:

- A self-referral occurs when a person applies for a care service themselves. Making an appointment to see your GP (family doctor) to discuss a health problem is an example of self-referral. Alternatively, phoning the NHS Direct service for advice and information or going to one of the NHS walk-in clinics are also ways of referring yourself to health care services.

- A professional referral occurs when a health or social care professional refers a person who has come to see them to another health or social care professional. An example of a professional referral occurs when a GP refers a patient to a hospital specialist (consultant) for further investigations or specialist treatment.

OVER TO YOU

For each of the following case studies identify:

(a) the client group involved;

(b) the type of referral(s) involved in each situation.

1 Mrs Arkwright is 78 years old and is frail. Her home carer noticed that she has a bad cough. The home carer rang Mrs Arkwright's GP, asking him to make a home visit.

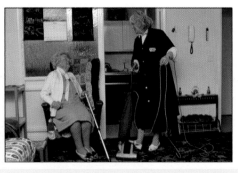

2 Rosie Abdi, a social worker, has received a phone call about a 3-year-old child who is being left alone during the day. The call came from a neighbour of the child's parents. Rosie has asked the family's GP to accompany her on a visit to the child's home.

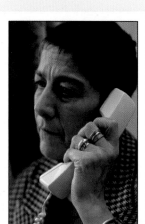

■ **Third-party referral** occurs when a person who is not a care professional applies for a care service on behalf of someone else. For example, if a woman telephoned the local social services department to request home care services for her mother, this would be a third-party referral.

Primary health care services are the front-line 'family doctor' or health centre services that are available in all local areas. People usually obtain primary health care services by self-referring or through a third-party referral. Everyone has a right to register with a GP and obtain primary health care services. If a person doesn't have a GP, their local health authority is expected to find them one within two working days.

Secondary health care services are more specialist hospital-based services. Some secondary health care services, such as accident and emergency (A&E) and sexually transmitted disease (STD) clinics, can be obtained by self-referral. However, most secondary health care services are obtained through a GP's professional referral. This applies to both inpatient care (the patient stays in hospital) and outpatient services (the patient lives at home and occasionally attends a hospital clinic).

To make a professional referral, a GP will contact a hospital consultant and request an appointment or an admission for their patient. The GP will tell the hospital how urgent the referral is.

3 Mr Ghupta, aged 35, has a long-term mental health problem. He goes to his local health centre or the local hospital's accident and emergency department when he feels unwell and needs treatment.

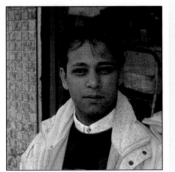

4 Elisha, aged 29, is five months pregnant. Her GP has made an appointment for her to have an ultrasound scan at the local hospital.

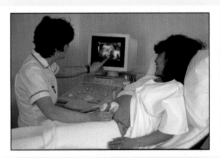

5 Jim has had a bad back for three days. His wife has made him an appointment with a private sector osteopath.

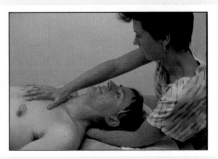

Barriers to health care services

There are occasions when people have a need for a care service, but they are unable to get it. Some of the most common 'barriers' to obtaining health care services are shown below

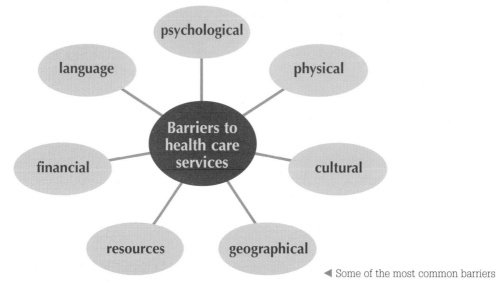

◄ Some of the most common barriers

Physical barriers

Physical barriers to health care services generally involve problems with the built environment. That is, some people can't get into the places where care services are provided, while others are unable to leave their own homes to go to the places where care is available. This is because the design of a building may prevent them entering or leaving. For example, a wheelchair user would be unable to obtain care services at a health centre if it had steps up to the front door and no other means of access. Other physical barriers, such as stairs or narrow corridors and doorways, occur within buildings and can prevent disabled and older people from using services.

Psychological barriers

Not everyone takes the same attitude towards their personal health and well-being. Some people avoid going to see their doctor for psychological reasons. This can be due to embarrassment, a lack of concern about their own health, or fear of the possible consequences. For example, the incidence of testicular cancer is higher than it should be because men are reluctant to conduct self-examinations or seek help early if they find anything unusual. You may know someone who is too scared to go to their doctor or dentist. This fear is a psychological barrier preventing them from getting the services that they may need.

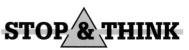

How do you think these physical barriers could be overcome to allow wheelchair users to gain access to care services?

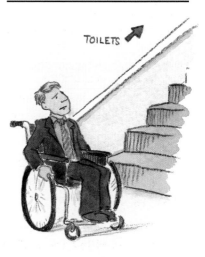

TOILETS

Financial barriers

Not all NHS services are free. For example, unless you are in an exempt group you will have to pay for prescriptions, eye tests and dental work. The cost of services can be a barrier to care for some people. For example, when free eye testing for people over 65 was withdrawn in 1989 there was a dramatic fall in the number of older people having eye tests. The British Medical Association claimed that this led to serious eye diseases and potential blindness not being detected. These free eye tests have now been reintroduced.

Geographical barriers

Health care services may be difficult to obtain if they are located several miles away from where people live. This is a particular problem for people who live in rural (country) areas. The problem is made even worse for people who rely on public transport. Sometimes people have to travel very long distances to obtain specialist treatments that aren't available in their own health district. The geographical location of services can act as a barrier to people getting the care they need. Health facilities that are difficult to get to are not likely to be used by people who do not have easy access to their own transport.

Cultural and language barriers

Health information is not always available in the languages that some people speak or in the formats needed by people who have eyesight or hearing problems. As a result, people can be deterred from using services because of the communication problems they face. In areas where there are large numbers of people from ethnic communities, health authorities try to ensure that language barriers are overcome by providing multi-language signs, interpreters and bilingual staff.

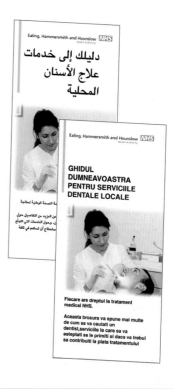

Resource barriers

The resources that organisations require before they can provide care services include:

- skilled staff
- buildings (including inpatient beds) and equipment
- money to pay the organisations' running costs and staff wages.

Care organisations may have staff shortages or not enough money to provide care services for people when they need them. This lack of resources can mean that people have to go on a waiting list for treatment. In this way, resource problems act as a barrier to care services.

Quick Questions

1 What kind of referral is used most often to obtain primary health care services?

2 Who does a GP need to contact to make a professional referral for specialist hospital services?

3 Explain how language barriers can prevent some people from obtaining the care services they need.

Access to social care

Access to both social care and early years services for children and adults can be by self-referral, third-party referral or professional referral. Referrals to statutory organisations, such as social services departments, will usually be dealt with by a duty social worker. It's their job to find out exactly what the situation is and what is needed.

Children's services

Local authority social services departments have clear procedures on how to deal with enquiries when a child may be at risk. In other cases involving children and families (where, for example, there are family relationship problems), a social worker will make an assessment to establish whether the children involved are in need. If so, as with child protection cases, services would be arranged to meet the children's needs.

Adult services

The key to adults obtaining social care services is an assessment of need. A person will receive social care services if they have an assessed need and they also meet the eligibility criteria that apply in the area where they live. The person carrying out the assessment will usually be a care co-ordinator or social worker.

OVER TO YOU

Try to find out what the eligibility criteria are for home help services in your local authority area.

Independent sector adult services

Much domiciliary, day and residential care is available directly from voluntary and private agencies. A self- or third-party referral will gain access to these services. Most agencies carry out their own assessments. The only eligibility criteria are that the person has the ability to pay and that the agency has the staff to supply the service.

Barriers to social care

The barriers to obtaining social care services are very similar to those that occur in health care. However three factors are more important than others.

■ **Psychological barriers**. Many people feel that there is a stigma (or sense of shame) attached to using social service departments, so they will avoid doing so, even if they have a clear need.

■ Finan...
means that ... **Adult services are means-tested.** This
assessed. Those wh... have to have their finances
by social services are elig... the financial limit imposed
have more money or savings th...rvices. People who
some or all of the cost of the service u...it have to pay
result, some ...d. As a
people can be
put off by the
costs involved or
by having to
disclose financial
information.

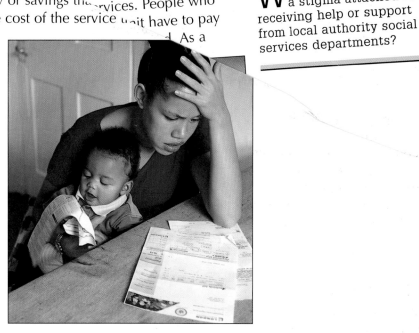

STOP & THINK

Why do you think there is a stigma attached to receiving help or support from local authority social services departments?

■ **Resource barriers.** Local authorities have to manage their
resources carefully. As a result they often increase the
eligibility criteria for services. For example, in the past
many local authorities would help someone who was
quite independent but who needed a home help to do
some cleaning and shopping for them. Nowadays, these
services are not available in many areas and someone
would have to need personal care on a daily basis before
they became eligible for a home help.

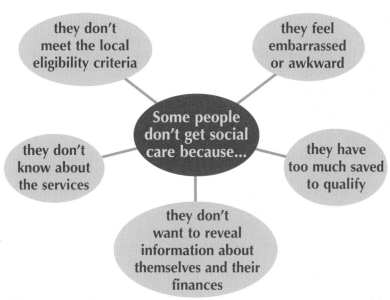

they don't meet the local eligibility criteria

they feel embarrassed or awkward

Some people don't get social care because...

they don't know about the services

they have too much saved to qualify

they don't want to reveal information about themselves and their finances

▲ Barriers to social care

Quick Questions

1 What is a means test?
2 Which type of care worker usually deals with a referral to a social services department?
3 Explain what has to happen before an adult can receive social care services from the local authority.

Early years services

For the most part, access to early years services is obtained by parents who apply direct to a private or voluntar~ ~er. A service provider, such as a private nursery or ~'ıs child will usually be offered a place if h~ afford the fees considered suitable, the parents a~following are a number of and there is a space availabl~ possible barriers to ac~~

- There is a ~~~age of state-run nursery education and day nurse~ places. Although there is no charge for state-run services in most cases, lack of places can prove to be the biggest barrier. This is an example of a **resource barrier**.

- Not all areas are well covered for pre-school provision, so location and transport difficulties may feature as significant problems. This is an example of a **geographical barrier**.

- Parents from a minority culture may struggle to find suitable care to meet their cultural needs, in terms of religious observance, language and so on. This is an example of a **cultural and language barrier**.

- The government has produced a National Childcare Strategy designed to increase the overall level of early years provision. However, for the most part parents will still be expected to pay for it. This can be a **financial barrier**.

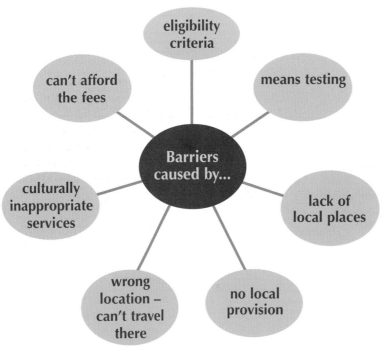

▲ Barriers to early years services

Build Your Learning

LEARNING POINTS

The following are the main points that you should have learnt from the previous seven pages.

- There are three main types of referral to care services – self-referral, professional and third party referral.

- A number of barriers can prevent people from obtaining the care they need.

- Barriers to obtaining care services can be classified as physical, psychological, financial, geographical, cultural or resource-based.

REVISION QUESTIONS

If you're confident that you understand the learning points and the key terms, try answering the revision questions below:

1 Identify two ways of obtaining primary health care services at your local GP practice.

2 Describe ways that resource factors can prevent people from obtaining the care they require.

3 Explain ways that cultural and language barriers can be overcome to help people obtain the care services they need.

The key question you should now be able to answer if you've understood the previous section is:

4 'How can people gain access to care services and what can prevent people from being able to use the services they need?'

KEY TERMS

You should know what the following terms mean:

- Referral (page 48)
- Self-referral (page 48)
- Professional referral (page 48)
- Third-party referral (page 49)
- Physical barriers (page 50)
- Psychological barriers (page 50)
- Geographical barriers (page 51)
- Financial barriers (page 51)
- Cultural or language barriers (page 51)
- Resource barriers (page 51)

If you're not sure or want to check your understanding, turn to the page number listed in the brackets.

INVESTIGATION IDEAS

1 Make a list of care services that you've used. Identify the method by which you gained access to, or obtained, each service.

2 Choose one or two local care organisations to investigate. Identify and describe the main barriers to access that exist for particular client groups. You should explain why members of these client groups might find the organisation's services difficult or impossible to use.

3 How are your local care organisations trying to overcome actual and potential barriers to access that affect their services? Collect newspaper articles, leaflets produced by the organisations and any other information you can find on this topic. Write a brief review of your findings.

Health, social care and early years organisations employ a large number of people. The NHS, for example, employs more people than any other organisation in Europe. Within the statutory health and social care sectors in the United Kingdom it is estimated that there are more than a million people in paid employment.

There is a wide variety of different jobs and specialist roles in health, social care and early years workplaces. Many of these jobs involve care workers working in teams in order to co-ordinate their efforts to help people. To simplify the range of care roles it is useful to consider the similarities and differences between:

- health care, social care and early years roles
- direct care workers and indirect care workers.

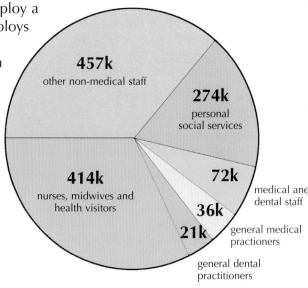

▲ NHS employees

Health, social care and early years roles

People employed as **health care workers** usually deal with individuals of all ages who have physical, medical-related problems such as a disease, injury or acute illness. **Social care workers** usually deal with people who are vulnerable and who have care needs that are mainly social, emotional or financial rather than medical in nature. **Early years workers** are usually employed in child care and early years education services for children under the age of eight.

Many care service users have both health and social care problems. This means that health care workers may need to provide social care as well as health care for a person. For example, a community psychiatric nurse who works with people experiencing mental health problems may need to offer his or her clients both health and social care.

Direct and indirect care workers

People who work in health, social care and early years services may have either a direct or an indirect care job. **Direct care** jobs involve providing one-to-one or face-to-face care to people in a practical way. Examples of direct care workers include nursery nurses and occupational therapists. **Indirect care** jobs involve providing support services. For example, people who work as receptionists, cleaners and porters have indirect care roles in health organisations. We are most likely to remember coming into contact with direct care workers such as nurses, doctors and social workers.

Areas of care work

Jobs in health and social care can also be grouped into a number of different areas of work. Some of the more familiar work areas are:

- medicine
- nursing
- social work or social care
- child care and early years education
- administration and support work.

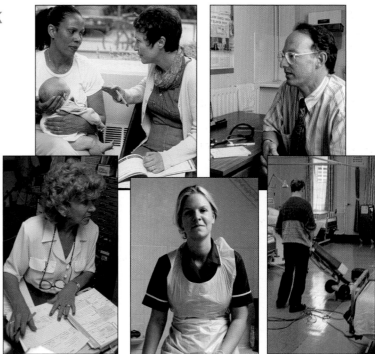

Within each area of work there are many specialist roles. Care workers tend to become more specialised as their careers progress. For example, within child care a person could begin his or her career as a nursery assistant, then qualify and work as a nursery nurse and, with further experience and training, go on to become a classroom teacher in primary education or a nursery manager for a local authority.

STOP & THINK

What kind of care work are you most interested in? Do you know what qualifications and experience are needed for this kind of work?

OVER TO YOU

1 Write a sentence that briefly describes what you believe is involved in each of the care jobs listed here. You could use careers booklets and computer databases to find out about occupational roles.

2 Reorganise the current list into three new lists headed 'Health jobs', 'Social care jobs' and 'Early years jobs'.

District nurse
Community psychiatric nurse
Care manager
Social worker
Nursery nurse
Housing advice worker
Health visitor

Residential social worker
Hospital manager
Gynaecologist
Chiropodist
Home care assistant
Childminder
Hostel manager
Surgeon

Quick Questions

1 According to official statistics, which care profession employs more care workers than any other?

2 Give two examples of indirect care jobs.

3 Explain the difference between a direct care job and an indirect care job.

Medicine

To qualify as a doctor it is necessary to have a degree in medicine. This involves attending a university medical school for five years to gain the basic academic knowledge and practical experience to pass this first stage of medical training. To gain entry to medical school an applicant usually needs at least five GCSEs and three A levels, or their equivalent, with very high grades. Most students enter medical school at the age of 18.

The work

After qualifying from university, he or she must then work for at least a year as a junior doctor in a hospital setting and rapidly gain experience of a range of diseases, illnesses and medical problems. Doctors spend most of their time examining patients, diagnosing their health problems and prescribing treatments. Doctors often work long hours and many work at weekends, in the evenings and at night to deal with the very large caseloads of patients they must see and treat. They also have to keep studying and must take professional examinations to become specialists (consultants) in areas of medicine such as surgery, general practice or psychiatry.

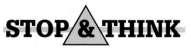

STOP & THINK

What kinds of skills do you think are needed by a doctor working in an accident and emergency department of a hospital?

CASE STUDY

Dr Lauren Campbell has worked as an anaesthetist at St Joseph's Hospital for three years. Her job is to anaesthetise patients and then to manage their airway and respiratory system safely while they are being treated or operated on. She works shifts to cover the 24-hour needs of the hospital and its patients. She works in the accident and emergency department and in the hospital's operating theatres. Dr Campbell works closely with other doctors and nursing staff as part of the team on call.

"You've got to be up to date with medical knowledge, careful and alert and confident to do my job."

CASE STUDY

Dr Bola Sarpei works as a GP at a health centre with three other GPs. She has a large and varied list of patients and sees them by appointment and at drop-in clinics between 8.30 a.m. and 6 p.m. each weekday. Dr Sarpei is able to diagnose and treat most of the illnesses that her patients come to her with, but she refers more complicated and serious cases to the local hospital. Dr Sarpei and her colleagues take it in turns to be on call one weekend in every four.

" Patience, good listening skills and calmness are the personal qualities needed to do my job. "

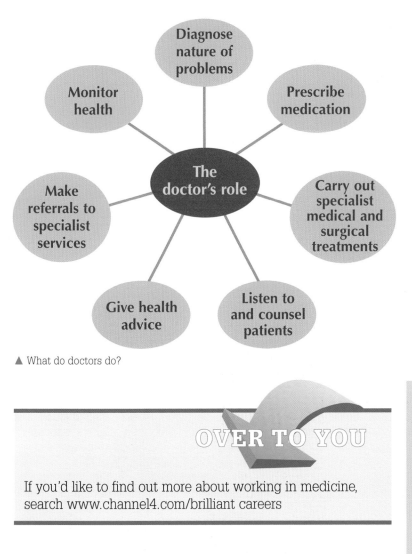

The doctor's role

- Diagnose nature of problems
- Prescribe medication
- Monitor health
- Carry out specialist medical and surgical treatments
- Make referrals to specialist services
- Listen to and counsel patients
- Give health advice

▲ What do doctors do?

OVER TO YOU

If you'd like to find out more about working in medicine, search www.channel4.com/brilliant careers

Quick Questions

1 What qualifications are needed to work as a doctor?

2 Name three tasks that doctors perform as part of their work.

3 What name is given to a highly qualified and experienced doctor who specialises in a particular area of hospital medicine?

Nursing

Nurses make up the largest group of care staff in the United Kingdom. There are approximately 345,000 qualified nurses working in a range of health care areas. There are four main branches of nursing: adult (also called general) nursing, children's nursing, learning disability nursing and mental health nursing. There are important differences in the type of training and work that these different professionally qualified nurses do. Additionally ,professionally qualified nurses also perform a different role to vocationally qualified health care support workers (also known as nursing assistants).

Registered nursing

Professionally qualified or registered nurses take an approved nurse training programme that lasts for three years and results in a registered nurse qualification. The minimum entry qualifications are passes in five GCSEs or equivalent. The minimum age for entry to nurse training is 17 and a half.

Once qualified, a registered nurse usually works as a staff nurse to gain experience and improve his or her practical skills. The day-to-day work that nurses do depends on the specialist area of care in which they work.

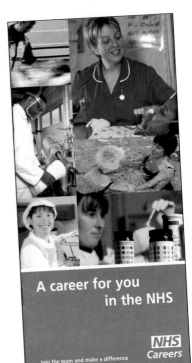

A career for you
in the NHS

NHS
Careers

Join the team and make a difference

CASE STUDY

Kathryn Williams is ward manager in the children's unit of a major teaching hospital. After qualifying as a registered general nurse fifteen years ago, she worked hard to become a ward manager. She has also worked in operating theatres and gained her BSc degree in nursing five years ago. Kathryn's work involves the day-to-day management of the unit. She has to plan the work rota to make sure enough staff are on duty, and must attend a variety of meetings about matters that affect the running of the unit, such as catering and cleaning. She also spends time supervising the nursing care of the children, meeting their parents and providing information and support for them and for other relatives, discussing the children's care and progress with the medical, physiotherapy and other care staff.

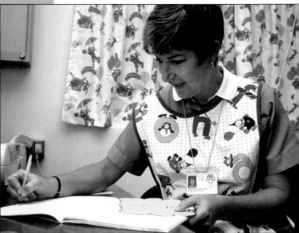

I have to be very well organised and need to be able to decide which tasks are a priority every day. Management skills are just as important as nursing skills in my job.

For example, mental health nurses spend a lot of time talking with service users and providing emotional support, whereas nurses working in accident and emergency spend more time treating people's wounds and injuries.

Generally, nurses spend a lot of time in very close contact with patients, providing a wide range of direct care and support. Nursing is often a physically and emotionally tiring job. Caring for people who are sick and dependent can involve carrying out tasks that are unpleasant and physically demanding, such as changing and remaking soiled beds. As well as carrying out their care role, nurses have to complete administrative work relating to patients and often have a role in training student nurses.

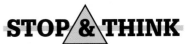
STOP & THINK

What skills do you think a registered nurse working with frail and confused older people would need? Would these skills be different to those needed to work with premature babies?

CASE STUDY

Sasha Edwards qualified as a registered mental health nurse two years ago. Sasha now works in a unit for frail older people who experience confusion and memory problems. Her day-to-day work can be very varied but includes tasks such as assessing individual patient's needs, providing direct care to help them to wash, dress and eat, and spending time talking and providing social and emotional support. Sasha also has to write in individual patient's notes and regularly attends meetings with doctors and other staff to discuss her patients' conditions and progress.

"*I like this kind of nursing because I have time to think about and really care for my patients. The pace isn't so fast as other types of nursing and I like to really get to know the people I care for.*"

Quick Questions

1 What qualifications are needed to train as a registered nurse?
2 Name the four branches of nursing.
3 What kind of skills does a nurse need to work as a ward manager?

OVER TO YOU

Find out about the real day-to-day work that nurses do by talking to somebody who works as a nurse. The school or college nurse may talk to your class about his or her work. Remember to prepare plenty of questions to ask them.

Health care support

Someone interested in direct care work can gain vocational training and experience as a **health care support worker**. Many health care support workers take an NVQ (National Vocational Qualification) course and gain their training and experience under the supervision of registered nurses. Health care support workers are employed in all areas of health care. They often have a lot of direct patient contact, assisting registered nurses and other care staff in providing care.

The role of a health care support worker is different to that of a registered nurse in a number of important ways.

- Health care support workers carry out most of the domestic tasks in a care setting, for example making beds.
- The physical care they provide relates to routine procedures such as lifting, washing, dressing and feeding clients.

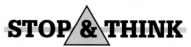

STOP & THINK

Which organisations employ health care support workers in your local area?

CASE STUDY

Rob Fitzgerald is 22 years old. He has worked as a health care support worker in a learning disabilities unit for the last five years. He works day and night shifts and provides direct care and support for the ten residents of the bungalow where he works. Rob helps the residents in different ways depending on their individual needs. Some people need help with personal care, such as going to the toilet, washing and dressing, while others need assistance when travelling to college or on social outings. All of the residents benefit from the relationships that they have developed with Rob. He is currently taking an NVQ level 2 in direct care and plans to develop his care and managerial skills. He hopes to work in day centres and progress to social work training later in his career.

" Most of the time I really like working in the bungalow and going out with the residents. It can be fun and it's practical work, which I like. It's all about the relationships you have with people and the way that you communicate with them really. "

■ Health care support workers carry out care planned by registered nurses.

Like nurses, health care support workers work day and night shifts and may also work at weekends. The minimum age requirement for health care support workers is 16. Personal maturity is one of the key factors that employers take into account when recruiting people to support worker posts.

Health Care Support Worker
37.5 hours per week
£10,034 per annum

Ref: HCSW 101

We are looking for motivated, enthusiastic people interested in working with older people. As a Health Care Support Worker you will work in a team of health care staff, have good communication skills and be well motivated. Care qualifications and previous experience desirable but not essential as training will be given to NVQ level 3.

Our aim is to provide a high standard of assessment and respite to patients who use our service.

For an application form and job description, please contact the Recruitment Office quoting the reference number for the post.

POSITION CARE ASSISTANT
Speciality: Adults with Learning Disabilities
Hours: 15–25 per week

Job Description: We require a cheerful and positive care assistant to work in a small residential unit for adults with learning disabilities. We offer good rates of pay, lots of fun and fantastic training and career opportunities. You must have a good sense of humour, be willing to learn, enjoy working with people and be practical.

We are looking for someone who will enjoy working as part of a team and who will relate to our residents as individuals. Ability to drive preferred, but this is not essential.

Quick Questions

1 What training qualification do many health care support workers take?

2 Explain how the work of a health care support worker is different to the work of a registered nurse.

3 What personal qualities do you think a person needs to work as a health care support worker?

OVER TO YOU

Find out more about the work of health care support workers by arranging to talk to a member of staff at a local hospital or nursing home. You might also be able to find information by looking at a careers website or by obtaining a job description when a vacancy for a health care support worker is advertised in your local paper.

Social work and social care

We said earlier that social care includes various forms of non-medical help for people who are vulnerable and in need of support. It may include forms of direct care such as counselling, or indirect help such as arranging housing or access to other support services. Social care services are provided by workers who have a variety of different job titles, such as project workers, community workers and social workers.

Social work

A social worker is a person who has gained a professional social work qualification (normally a Diploma in Social Work), and who has experience of working with clients with social, financial and emotional problems. Diploma in Social Work courses are available in further and higher education colleges. Applicants usually need a minimum of A level or other advanced level qualifications, and some social care experience. Because it is difficult and stressful work that requires maturity and life experience, most social work courses have a minimum entry age of 21.

Most professionally qualified social workers are employed as field social workers. This means that they have a caseload of people they work with in community and institutional settings. Some social workers specialise in working with particular types of clients, such as those in child protection work or psychiatric social work, whereas others operate as non-specialised social workers and see people referred to them with various problems. Field social workers specialise in the provision of social work services. Some social workers work as care co-ordinators or care managers and specialise in assessing clients' needs and purchasing care packages for them (see page 36).

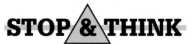

STOP & THINK

Can you think of reasons why social work is sometimes a difficult and stressful job?

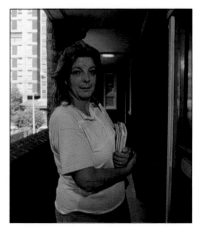

▲ Social workers need a wide range of skills and personal qualities

◀ What do social workers do?

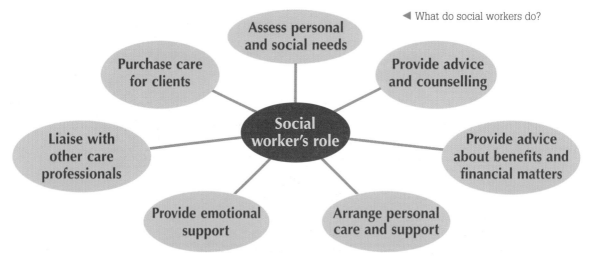

Social worker's role
- Assess personal and social needs
- Provide advice and counselling
- Provide advice about benefits and financial matters
- Arrange personal care and support
- Provide emotional support
- Liaise with other care professionals
- Purchase care for clients

Social care

There is a range of vocationally qualified and non-qualified people who also work in social care settings in a support capacity. Like health care support workers, social care support workers now tend to have NVQ training gained through experience. They work under the supervision of qualified social workers, often providing practical help and support for clients that requires direct client contact. Social care support workers may work in:

- domiciliary (home) care
- residential care
- day care.

Social care workers may work a variety of different shift patterns. Day care workers tend to work 9a.m. to 5p.m., Monday to Friday; domiciliary care workers may work at any time of the day from early morning to late evening; residential social care workers may work day and night shifts and weekends. The minimum age for entry into this type of care work is 16. As with health care support worker posts, employers look for people with personal maturity and some life experience that gives them the ability to help and support others.

Quick Questions

1 What qualifications are needed to train as a social worker?

2 What kinds of care services do domiciliary care workers provide?

3 With which two client groups are domiciliary care workers most likely to work?

CASE STUDY

Denise Mann is employed as a home carer by a Local Authority. She works a shift system that includes days, nights and weekend work. Denise has taken an NVQ level 2 course and has been on food hygiene and lifting and handling courses. She visits up to six different older people in their homes each day. She helps them to wash and dress and prepares breakfast or an evening drink for them. Denise enjoys the practical side of her job and feels that it is important to be well organised and understanding to do her job well.

My job is quite tiring but I think it's important to help people. I enjoy the practical work and think of my clients as friends as well.

OVER TO YOU

Find out more about the role of a social worker by looking at either the General Social Care Council (GSCC) courses website www.swap.ac.uk or www.socialworkcareers.co.uk They both publicise social work training. You might also be able to get information by looking at other careers websites or by obtaining a job description when a vacancy for a social worker is advertised in your local paper.

Child care and early years education

There is a wide range of care roles and career opportunities in child care and early years education. Child care and early years workers may have qualifications or may gain work because of their own experience in bringing up children. Many nursery, playgroup and classroom assistants now also undertake NVQ training, for example, to add new knowledge and skills to their child care work.

Child care and early years work involves plenty of busy, hands-on activities with children. Care workers in this area are responsible for the safety and development of the children in their care. Some early years workers specialise in working with children who have physical or sensory impairments (see page 38), whereas others specialise in working with children who have learning difficulties. Some of the similarities and differences in the qualifications and roles of different child care and early years workers are described below.

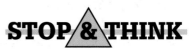

STOP & THINK

How many local organisations can you think of where people are employed as child care and early years workers?

Nursery nursing

A qualified nursery nurse has achieved a qualification such as an NNEB or BTEC Diploma in Nursery Nursing. Nursery nurses are employed in private and local authority nurseries, usually providing direct care and education for children under five.

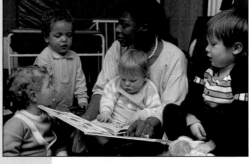

Playgroup assistant

People who work as assistants in playgroups and nurseries work under the supervision of a nursery nurse or another experienced playgroup worker. Many carers take NVQ qualifications to improve their knowledge and skills. The minimum age requirement is 16 with no specific qualifications required to gain entry to playgroup work.

Play specialist

Play specialists work with children in hospital. Their role is to use play as a way of developing children's practical and communication skills at a time in their lives when ordinary school life and opportunities to play with other children are limited by their illnesses or disabilities.

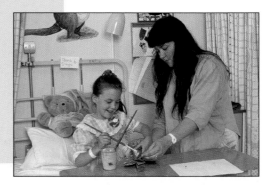

Early years teacher

Nursery and infant teachers work in state and private primary schools. They must have a degree to obtain a post. They work with groups of children, planning and assessing learning activities for them, often using play to achieve this. Early years teachers work school hours but often also work at home to prepare and mark work and do their record keeping.

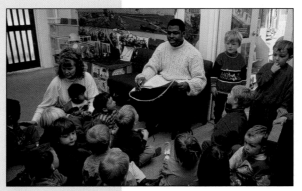

Classroom assistant

Classroom assistants are not qualified teachers. They assist the teacher with practical activities, such as setting up the classroom and supervising children on outings. They also help children with basic care tasks, such as changing their clothes and going to the toilet when they are unable to do this for themselves. Classroom assistants can take specialist courses and NVQs to improve their skills. They work school hours.

Registered childminder

Childminders work in their own home looking after one or more children, usually in office or other working hours when the children's parents are working. Childminders must be registered with their local authority and must be able to offer the facilities and experience needed to provide a good standard of care. The minimum age requirement for registered childminders is set down by the local authority and is usually 21.

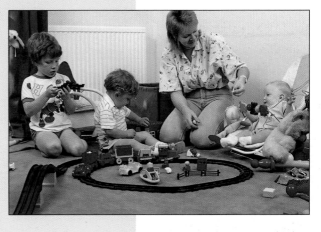

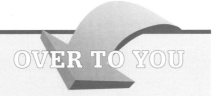
OVER TO YOU

Colleges of further education provide many child care and early years courses for both full- and part-time students. Find out what's available at your local college by looking at their website or by obtaining a prospectus of courses.

Quick Questions

1 What qualifications do nursery nurses usually have?
2 What skills do you think are needed to work with children under eight?
3 Describe how the work of a nursery nurse is different to that of an early years teacher.

Administration, management and ancillary jobs

Health and social care organisations employ a wide range of support staff who carry out the administrative, management and ancillary jobs that are essential for all organisations and direct care workers to work efficiently.

Administrative work

Administrative work includes secretarial and clerical jobs such as typing, filing, record keeping and wages calculations. Information technology, accountancy, typing and customer care courses are all available to administrative workers either as NVQ courses through colleges or through training departments within care organisations.

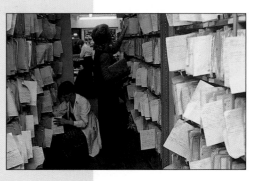

Management work

Management work involves taking responsibility for the effective and efficient running of various aspects of a care organisation. People who work as managers may have specialist qualifications in the area in which they are working, such as medical laboratory science, or an additional management qualification and experience gained through working in various posts. Managers have more power and responsibility than administrative staff and are often responsible for a group of staff and a department. Managers usually work office hours, Monday to Friday. They may have a variety of qualifications including NVQs, degrees and diplomas in different areas of management.

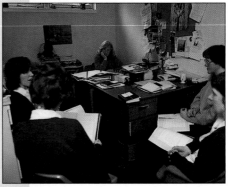

Ancillary work

Ancillary work covers areas needed to keep a care organisation running effectively, such as catering, cleaning and maintenance. People employed as ancillary staff may have vocational qualifications appropriate to the area in which they work, for example catering or electrical work. Many obtain their jobs because of their previous experience and their practical skills. Ancillary staff work a variety of shift patterns. Some work office hours while others work at night and at weekends to keep the care services operating.

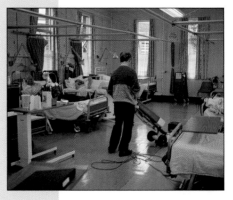

CASE STUDY

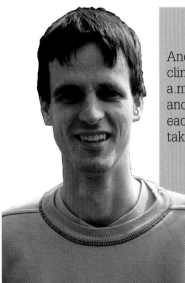

Andy Johnson works as a domestic cleaner in an outpatient clinic attached to the hospital. He works five days a week, 5 a.m. to 8 a.m. He is responsible for cleaning the floors, desks and other surfaces, and generally he tidies the department each morning before other people arrive. Andy is currently taking an NVQ level 2 in Cleaning.

"My job is very physical. You need to be fit and pay attention to doing things right. I am well organised and can work on my own but I prefer to be part of a team. We work hard and do a good job together."

CASE STUDY

Barbara Henry is the facilities manager at St Joseph's Hospital. She is responsible for the safe and efficient running of the catering, laundry, portering and gardening services that operate behind the scenes at St Joseph's. Barbara works with the staff in each of the areas mentioned, holding daily meetings to discuss staffing and operational issues. She also liaises with other managers responsible for the direct care and financial aspects of running the hospital. She works mainly between 9 a.m. to 5 p.m., but she can be contacted outside of office hour to sort out problems.

"My working day is very busy. I have a lot of meetings to attend and need to make sure that I see the support staff regularly. My job requires a range of business and management skills but I think that being a good communicator and problem-solver is the key to it."

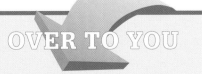

OVER TO YOU

Find out about the work roles of receptionists and porters. What do each of these jobs involve and why are they essential to the running of hospital care services?

Quick Questions

1 Name two jobs that involve administrative work.
2 Explain why care organisations need to employ a range of ancillary workers.
3 Explain why a hospital manager is an indirect rather than a direct care worker.

Communication skills

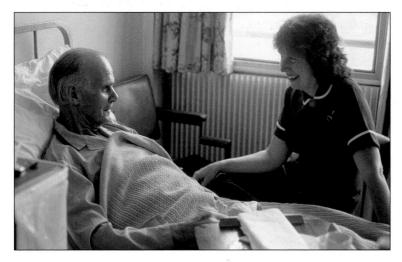

◄ What communication skills is this nurse using?

Care workers use a range of different communication skills during their working day (or night). These include listening and various types of verbal (talking) skills, as well as touch and forms of body language. A care worker has to use their communication skills when they:

- carry out an assessment of an individual's care needs
- give or receive information about the care they provide
- provide emotional support to a client or family member.

Communication is about making contact with others and being understood. It involves sending and receiving messages. We all communicate, or send messages, continuously.

Types of communication

Most of the communication between care workers and clients occurs through a combination of verbal (speaking) and non-verbal (body language) methods.

Verbal communication occurs when one person speaks and another person listens. Care workers need a range of verbal communication skills to:

- respond to clients' questions
- find out about a client's problems
- contribute to team meetings
- break bad news
- provide support to others
- deal with problems and complaints.

Effective verbal communication involves a two-way process of speaking and listening. Listening is much harder than speaking! As well as communicating through speech, we all communicate in a variety of non-verbal ways.

Non-verbal communication is often referred to as body language. It involves using our bodies and appearance to communicate in various ways. For example, a care worker's behaviour and demeanour sends messages to clients and colleagues about how much they care for and respect them. Similarly, a client's body language may tell a care worker that they are experiencing pain or are uncomfortable even when they say everything's OK. Body language provides a continual channel of communication for others to read. Important features of non-verbal communication include:

- facial expression
- eye-contact
- gesture
- posture
- proximity and touch.

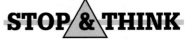

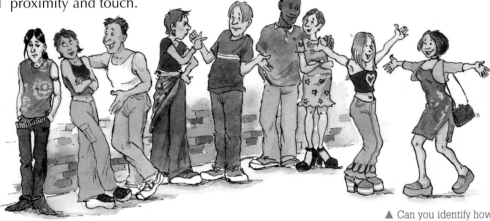

▲ Can you identify how these people are communicating non-verbally?

Using communication skills in care work

Care workers use verbal and non-verbal communication skills in a variety of ways. For example, care workers need to have good observation skills to learn about their clients. This is important in carrying out assessments of clients' needs and in checking on progress during or after treatment. Interviewing clients and their relatives is often a part of assessment. This relies on the care worker having the ability to ask questions and listen carefully to what the client says. Effective written skills are required to write up the assessments so that they can be understood by colleagues.

Care workers have to attend many meetings with colleagues in which they discuss and report on clients' problems and progress. These meetings may occur on a daily basis, where care workers use their verbal and listening skills to update each other on clients' daily progress. Groups of care workers may also meet to hold a case conference or another formal meeting to review a client's situation. In both of these types of meetings written notes may be made to provide a record of the meeting and of the client's progress.

Quick Questions

1 Name the two main types of communication.

2 What are the two things that people have to do during verbal communication?

3 Describe two ways that care workers might use their communication skills in a care setting.

Effective communication

Communication with clients is most effective when it occurs within a supportive care relationship. These care relationships don't just happen, they have to be created and maintained. People communicate most effectively when they feel relaxed, when they are able to empathise with the other person, and when they experience warmth and genuineness in the relationship.

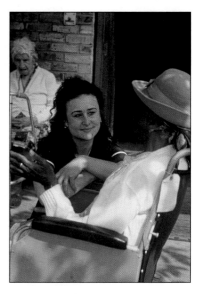

- **Empathy** means the ability to sense the feelings of others, to be able to put yourself in their shoes and feel what they feel. It involves trying to appreciate how they see and experience the world. Being empathic improves a care worker's ability to communicate.

- Expressing **warmth** is important. It makes a person feel accepted and secure, and builds trust.

- **Genuineness** involves being yourself and communicating with honesty and integrity. Care workers who are genuine avoid being authoritarian, defensive or emotionally detached. Genuineness also involves making sure that verbal and non-verbal messages match or support each other, being consistent in how you approach clients and being open and honest with people.

Care workers who build effective relationships with people in care settings treat them with respect and dignity and as individuals.

Quick Questions

1 How does someone who is genuine behave?

2 Explain why empathy is an important part of a care worker's communication skills.

3 What effect might bad communication have on a person receiving care?

The benefits of effective communication

For care workers

1 Helps carers to give and receive information that is relevant to their clients' care and well-being.

2 Enables care workers to express trust, acceptance, understanding and support.

3 Allows carers to identify and meet the individual needs of each client.

4 Enables carers to identify and support clients' abilities and reduces dependency.

For clients

1 Enables clients to feel secure and respected as individuals at times when they are physically and emotionally vulnerable.

2 Co-operation, involvement and partnership in a care relationship require open and supportive communication.

3 Empowers clients by allowing them to express their needs, worries and wishes.

4 Clients need to maintain their sense of identity while receiving care. This can only be achieved if they have opportunities to express themselves and be understood by their carers.

OVER TO YOU

Carry out some role-play activities with a colleague in your class to demonstrate and improve your communication skills. Take it in turns to be an interviewer and an interviewee and then assess the strengths and weaknesses of each other's verbal, listening and body-language skills.

Build Your Learning

LEARNING POINTS

The following are the main points that you should have learnt from the previous 17 pages.

- Jobs in care can be described as health, social or early years roles.
- Direct care workers usually specialise in a particular area of care work, such as medicine, nursing, social work or childcare.
- Indirect care workers usually specialise in support roles such as management, accountancy or administration.
- Care workers need to develop and use a range of communication skills effectively in their day to day work. Good communication skills are vital for good client care.

KEY TERMS

You should know what the following terms mean:

- Health care workers (page 56)
- Social care workers (page 56)
- Early years workers (page 56)
- Direct care (page 56)
- Indirect care (page 56)
- Junior doctor (page 58)
- Consultant (page 58))
- Registered Nurse (page 60)
- Health care support worker (page 62)
- Diploma in Social Work (page 64)
- Verbal communication (page 70)
- Non-verbal communication (page 71)
- Empathy (page 72)
- Warmth (page 72)
- Genuineness (page 72)

If you're not sure or want to check your understanding, turn to the page number listed in the brackets.

REVISION QUESTIONS

If you're confident that you understand the learning points and the key terms, try answering the revision questions below.

1 Identify two direct and two indirect care jobs that people carry out in hospitals.

2 Describe ways in which care workers use verbal communication skills in their work with service users.

3 Explain why care workers should try to make empathy, warmth and genuineness part of their communication with service users and their families.

The key question you should now be able to answer if you've understood the previous section is:

4 'What does care work involve and what skills do care practitioners need to perform their work roles?'

INVESTIGATION IDEAS

1 Research the care profession or job role in which you're most interested. You should be able to find out more information by carrying out an internet search, by looking at careers booklets and databases and by talking to people who already do the job. Produce an in-depth profile of the role covering entry routes (ways of getting in), what the work really involves and ways of developing a career in this area of work.

2 Find a care professional whose job you're interested in and arrange a work placement or job shadowing placement with them. Produce a 'Day in the life' account of what they actually do and what their job involves. Remember to ask their permission before doing this.

3 Collect newspaper and magazine articles about the work of health and social care professionals. You might also like to watch TV programmes about this area of work. Make a note of how they present the work of care professionals. Do they present it accurately or do the media stereotype care workers?

What is a value base?

Value base is an odd-sounding phrase that actually means something quite simple. If you value something, you feel that it is important or worthwhile. For example, you probably expect your friends to be honest with you and to respect your feelings. Why? Because you probably believe that telling the truth and showing respect are the right ways to behave and that telling lies to friends and disrespecting them are wrong. Care values are beliefs about the right ways to treat patients or clients. When all the values are put together, they make up a value base.

Care workers are expected to understand and put into practice a number of important care values in their work with people. For example, they are expected to understand why it is important to avoid discriminating against people and to put this into practice when they deal with people from different backgrounds. You would probably expect your GP (family doctor) to say 'I try to treat all people equally, whoever they are', or your counsellor to say 'It's important to keep the things my client talks to me about confidential'.

Examples of the values that care workers are expected to understand and put into practice include:

- promoting anti-discriminatory practice
- maintaining confidentiality of information
- promoting and supporting individuals' rights (to dignity, independence and safety)
- acknowledging individuals' personal beliefs and identity
- protecting individuals from abuse
- promoting effective communication and relationships
- providing individualised care.

Why use care values?

Care values are now seen as an essential part of the work of all care practitioners. Care professionals who need to be on a register of qualified practitioners before they are allowed to practise (registered nurses, physiotherapists and doctors, for example) are expected to follow the codes of practice and guidelines issued by their professional bodies. These codes of practice and guidelines express the care values of the profession. Breaking them or not following them will result in a practitioner being 'struck off' the professional register. This will prevent them from working in their care profession.

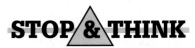

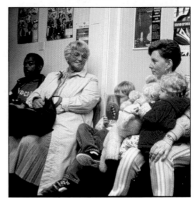

How do you expect care workers to behave towards you when you use care services?

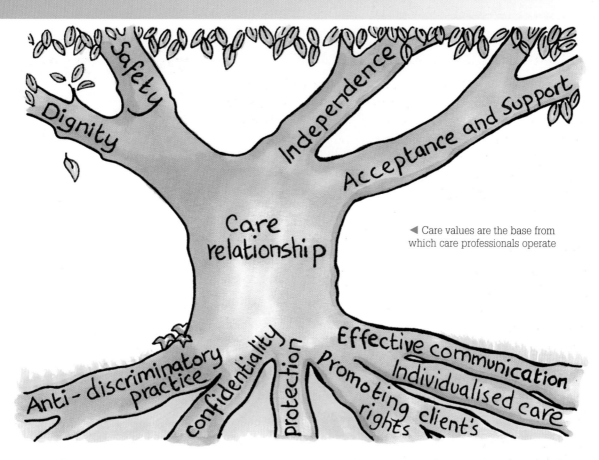

Care values are the base from which care professionals operate

Applying care values

Care values are used to protect the interests of all service users. Guidelines and codes of practice are produced to ensure that all service users are well treated and that their health and care needs are uppermost in the minds of care workers. This can sometimes lead to difficult decisions having to be made about what is in a person's best interest.

When people know and accept that they have care needs, they will usually welcome the help and support offered by care workers. However, there are situations where people don't know or don't accept that they require help and support. Care workers may then have to intervene even though the client says they don't need help. For example, some forms of mental illness affect a person's ability to know the difference between what is and what isn't real or true. The same thing can happen when children or young people are seen by care workers to be at risk and in need of protection, despite protests from their parents or carers that this is not the case. In these situations care workers have the difficult job of having to make a decision about what is in the best interest of the child and any other people who may be affected by their decision. The care worker must make an assessment of the risks involved in doing nothing, as much as those involved in doing something.

Quick Questions

1 Identify three important values that are applied by care workers.

2 Explain what a care value is.

3 What is a care value base?

Promoting anti-discriminatory practice

Unfair discrimination occurs when individuals or groups of people are treated differently, unequally and unfairly in comparison to others. For example, an employer who refused to interview candidates under the age of 25 for a nursery manager post because 'in my experience, younger people are not good at accepting responsibility', would be unfairly discriminating against this group of people .

The main cause of unfair discrimination is prejudice – having negative or hostile feelings, ideas and attitudes towards other people. Prejudice usually involves making judgements about people on the basis of untrue, ill-informed or exaggerated feelings, ideas and attitudes. When people are prejudiced they are often prejudiced against specific groups of people. In the United Kingdom, some of the social groups that tend to experience unfair discrimination include:

- minority ethnic groups
- minority religious groups
- women
- lesbians and gay men
- older people
- the learning- and physically disabled
- people with mental health problems.

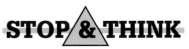

STOP & THINK

Why do you think members of these particular groups experience unfair discrimination?

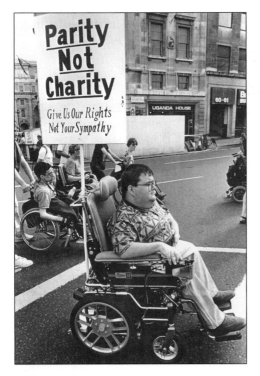

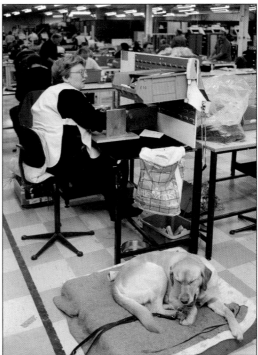

Anti-discriminatory care practice

Care workers who take an anti-discriminatory approach are:

- aware of the different forms of unfair discrimination that can occur in care settings
- sensitive to the ethnic and social background and cultural needs of each individual for whom they provide care
- prepared to actively challenge and work towards reducing the unfair discrimination experienced by the people for whom they provide care.

People experience unfair discrimination because of their race or colour (racism), gender (sexism), age (ageism), disability (disablism), sexuality (homophobia), religion or health status. Carers should never unfairly discriminate against people. Wherever they receive care, all patients and clients are entitled to non-discriminatory treatment. However, anti-discriminatory practice does not just mean treating everybody the same. It also means challenging and reducing any form of unfair discrimination that might be experienced by individuals.

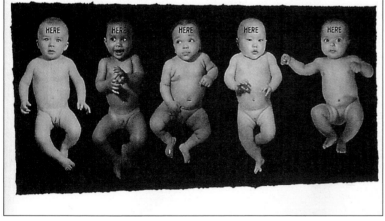

THERE ARE LOTS OF PLACES IN BRITAIN WHERE RACISM DOESN'T EXIST.

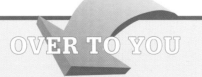

OVER TO YOU

Find out more about racial discrimination by looking at the Commission for Racial Equality website (www.cre.org.uk). Find out more about sexual discrimination by looking at the Equal Opportunities Commission website www.eoc.gov.uk.

Quick Questions

1 Name three groups who often experience unfair discrimination in the United Kingdom.

2 What is the main cause of all forms of unfair discrimination?

3 In your own words, explain what care workers do if they take an anti-discriminatory approach to their work.

Maintaining the confidentiality of information

Effective relationships are based on the trust that people have in each other. If you cannot trust another person with your thoughts and feelings you are not likely to develop a strong or deep relationship with them.

Confidentiality in care work

The care relationship is based on trust and particularly on the need for care workers to maintain confidentiality whenever possible. Confidentiality is an important value in care work. However, sometimes decisions are made to disclose information that breaks client confidentiality. These decisions should never be taken lightly and each situation must be thought through individually.

There are times when it is important to keep confidences and information that you have about clients to yourself. For example, if a child at the nursery where you do your work placement swore at you and misbehaved one afternoon, or an elderly resident at a nursing home refused to bathe after wetting herself, you would be breaching confidentiality to reveal these things to your friends. You should not breach confidentiality in situations where service users have a right to privacy or where their comments or behaviour do not cause anybody harm or break the law. Where care workers gossip or talk publicly about events or issues that happen at work they are betraying the trust that service users and colleagues put in them.

There may, however, be occasions when a care worker must reveal what they have been told, or seen for themselves, to a more senior person at work. When service users request that what they say is kept secret, this can be overridden if:

- what they reveal involves them breaking the law or planning to do so
- they say that they intend to harm themselves or another person
- they reveal information that can be used to protect another person from harm.

If an offence is committed that could have been prevented by the care worker revealing the confidence, they could be brought to court to face charges. Care workers should never promise service users that what they say will be absolutely confidential. They should explain that there are times when they may have to share information with their colleagues and other authorities.

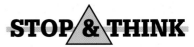

STOP & THINK

Do you think that a GP (family doctor) should tell a teenager's parents if she requested to be prescribed the contraceptive pill?

Quick Questions

1 What does keeping something confidential mean?
2 Why is confidentiality important in care work?
3 When should a care worker break confidentiality?

The following situations all involve decisions about confidentiality. For each one explain:

- why confidentiality may be important to the client;
- the dilemma facing the care worker;
- whether you would break confidentiality and why.

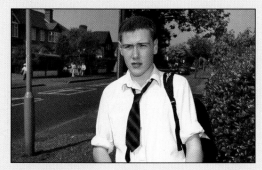

- Darren has an appointment with the school nurse for a BCG booster injection. He's worried about it making him ill. He says that he's just taken some Ecstasy and pleads with the nurse not to tell anyone.

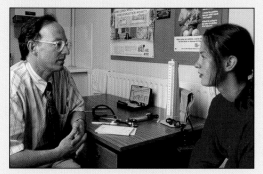

- Jennifer goes to her GP for contraceptive pills. She asks her GP not to tell her parents. She is 14 years old.

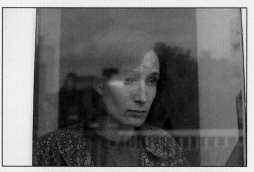

- Eileen has terminal cancer. She tells her district nurse that she's had enough of living and is going to end her own life tomorrow. She says it's her choice and asks the district nurse not to interfere.

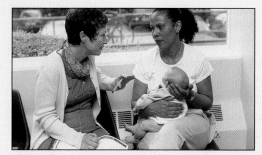

- Yasmin tells her new health visitor that her boyfriend is violent and is beating her. She asks the health visitor not to say anything as she is frightened of what might happen. Yasmin and her boyfriend have a 3-month-old baby.

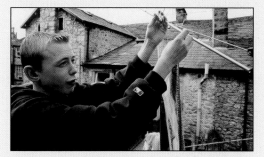

- Lee turns up at a hostel for the homeless. He says that he has run away from home because his father has been beating him. He asks the social worker not to contact his family. He is 16 years old.

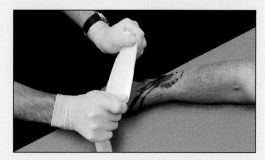

- A man with a stab wound arrives at the hospital casualty department. He won't give his name and asks the nurse not to phone the police. He says that he will leave if the nurse does. He is bleeding heavily.

Promoting and supporting individuals' rights

The relationship that a care worker develops with a service user is the cornerstone of all the work that they do as a care provider. In the previous section we looked at the need for trust in the care relationship. This is the basis of the care relationship. In addition to this, good care relationships also promote and support service users' rights to have their dignity respected, make their own decisions, and have their safety and security protected while they are receiving care.

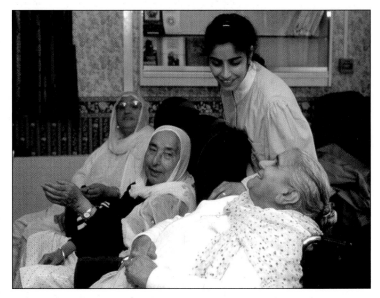

It is good practice on the part of carers and care organisations to give service users choices about their care and to encourage them to make decisions about this themselves. Ideally, care workers and service users should develop partnerships in which the service user feels equally involved. This kind of relationship is empowering because service users are seen as:

■ individuals with rights and choices appropriate to their age and needs

■ deserving of respect, regardless of their personal or social characteristics.

Acknowledging people's personal beliefs and identity

Acknowledging people's personal beliefs and identity means that care workers should try to communicate that they accept people for who they are and what they believe. Care workers may not always share the beliefs and lifestyle of the people they care for, but should still show that they accept their client's individuality. For example, if you care for people who have different religious beliefs and practices to your own, you should give them the opportunity to practise their faith and celebrate their religious festivals at times when this is important to them.

Protecting individuals from abuse

Many people who use care services are at a vulnerable point in their life and put a lot of trust in care workers to provide

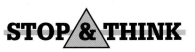

Can you think of any religions or ways of life that result in people having special dietary needs?

them with the help and support they need. Some groups of service users, including children, older people, disabled people and people with mental health problems, are vulnerable to exploitation and abuse by others.

This can be because of the problems they have or because they are less powerful and are easily influenced by unscrupulous people. As a result, many people who need or who are receiving care face a greater risk of experiencing a form of abuse (physical, emotional or sexual, for example).

Protecting service users from potential abuse is something that all care workers should feel is important. Care workers should assess the relationships that their clients have with other people for any signs of abuse and should always act to prevent this occurring or stop it happening when they become aware of it.

Promoting effective communication and relationships

Empowering relationships depend on care workers using their communication skills effectively in their interactions with others. Being sensitive to what other people are saying, thinking and feeling, treating them with respect, and protecting their dignity and rights, are all features of empowering care practice. To be able to do these things, care workers need to be sensitive to the spoken and unspoken communication of their clients. They also need to be aware of how they themselves think, feel and behave in their interactions with clients.

Looking after people is only one part of care work. On its own, this approach may result in a person becoming dependent on their carer. Good care practice also involves the carer working to promote the independence and development of the individuals for whom they provide care.

Providing individualised care

Care workers often provide care for people who have similar problems and needs. However, rather than treating everyone the same they should provide care that meets each person's individual needs. This involves assessing particular needs, identifying and acknowledging personal beliefs and preferences and working to provide care in ways that best suits the individual. Where this doesn't happen, people complain that care services are impersonal and don't meet their individual needs. They start to feel as though they're treated as a patient, not as a person, and that their right to make decisions and have choices is taken away. Individualised care is valued by care workers because it respects the rights and dignity of care service users as individuals and as people.

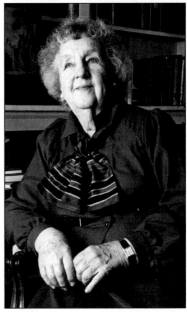

Virginia Henderson (1897–1996) was an important nursing figure in the twentieth century.

> *I say that the nurse does for others what they would do for themselves if they had the strength, the will, and the knowledge. But I go on to say that the nurse makes the patient independent of him or her as soon as possible.*

Virginia Henderson's classic definition of nursing.

Quick Questions

1 Explain why care service users need to be protected from abuse.

2 What is individualised care?

3 What can happen if service users don't receive individualised care

Codes of practice, policies and procedures

To help ensure that care workers respect clients' rights, codes of practice, policies and procedures have been developed by professional organisations and employers. These are now used in all care settings.

Codes of practice

A code of practice is a document that outlines an agreed way of working and dealing with specified situations. Codes of practice aim to reflect and set a standard for good practice in care settings. A number of codes of practice have been developed for care workers such as registered nurses, occupational therapists and physiotherapists, social workers and nursery staff. Codes of practice establish the general principles and standards for care workers and should always refer to equality of opportunity.

Policies and procedures

A policy is different to a code of practice in that it tells care workers how they should approach specific issues in a particular care setting. For example, most care homes will have a policy on confidentiality. This will explain in detail how this issue is dealt with in the particular home. Policies should promote equal treatment and equality of opportunity for everyone likely to be affected by them.

A procedure describes the way that staff in a particular care setting are expected to deal with an issue or activity in which they are involved. For example, care homes for older people usually have written procedures that describe how to deal with a situation where a resident goes missing from the home. The procedure will set out in detail the steps that the staff should take in trying to locate the person and report them missing to the relevant authorities.

Policies and procedures should always incorporate the main values of the care profession. They should ensure that service users' rights are respected and that activities are always carried out in the service users' best interests.

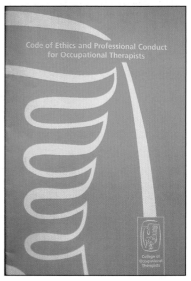

▲ The code of practice for occupational therapists

Build Your Learning

LEARNING POINTS

The following are the main points that you should have learnt from the previous nine pages.

- Care workers base their practice on a number of important values. These are ideas about the ways that care service users should be treated.

- Care workers use care values both to protect service users' interests and also to promote high standards of practice.

- Care values are incorporated into codes of practice and organisational policies and procedures.

- Codes of practice, policies and procedures provide care workers with guidance and sets of rules for how they should approach specific situations (protecting confidentiality of information, for example) and care practice generally.

KEY TERMS

You should know what the following terms mean:

- Care values (page 74)
- Value base (page 74)
- Prejudice (page 76)
- Anti-discriminatory practice (page 76)
- Prejudice (page 76)
- Confidentiality (page 78)
- Empowerment (page 80)
- Individualised care (page 81)
- Code of practice (page 82)
- Policy (page 82)
- Procedure (page 82)

If you're not sure or want to check your understanding, turn to the page number listed in the brackets.

REVISION QUESTIONS

If you're confident that you understand the learning points and the key terms, try answering the revision questions below.

1 Identify three care values that all care workers should try to use in their care practice.

2 Describe ways in which a care worker can ensure that confidentiality is maintained on behalf of a service user.

3 Explain the purpose of a code of practice.

The key question you should now be able to answer if you've understood the previous section is:

4 'What values do care workers promote through their work?'

INVESTIGATION IDEAS

1 Obtain a copy of a code of practice used by nurses, social workers or any other care professional. A local care organisation or care practitioner may provide you with a copy. Alternatively, carry out an internet search and look at the websites of the main regulatory bodies for these professions (for example, for nursing try *www.nmc-uk.org*). You may be able to print a copy their code of practice from the site. Using this code of practice, identify the main points in the code and check if it refers to all the values that we've covered.

2 At your work placement, ask a qualified care worker or somebody in charge, about the policies, procedures and codes of practice that affect their work. Make summary notes of what they tell you.

3 How do care service users expect to be treated by care workers? Carry out a brief survey of your friends and family to identify which of the care values we've covered they feel are the most important.

Promoting health and wellbeing

This unit is about the different ways that people think about and try to achieve personal health and wellbeing. You will learn about:

- definitions of health and wellbeing
- common factors affecting health and wellbeing and the different effects they can have across the human life span
- the methods used to measure an individual's physical health
- ways of promoting and supporting health improvement for an individual or for a small group.

Health and wellbeing are terms that you should understand. It is important that you are able to identify what good physical health involves and that you have an understanding of some of the measures of health used by care workers. You should be able to appreciate and explain the effects of a person's lifestyle on his or her health and wellbeing. Learning about different lifestyle practices that may put an individual's health at risk, and about the ways in which health promotion information can be provided will be of benefit if you choose to work with people in care situations.

The material in this unit covers Unit 2, Promoting health and wellbeing, of the GCSE Health and Social Care award.

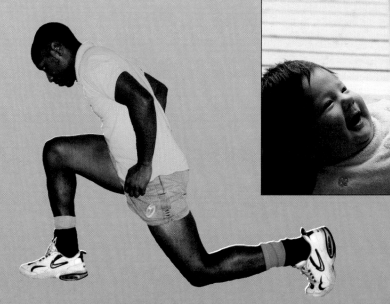

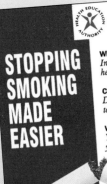

STOPPING SMOKING MADE EASIER

HEALTH EDUCATION AUTHORITY

Where to get help
Includes a telephone helpline

Checklist
Do you really want to stop?

Will power
You have more than you think

Planning ahead
The simple secret of success

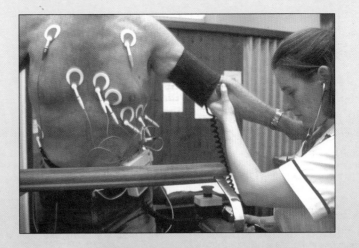

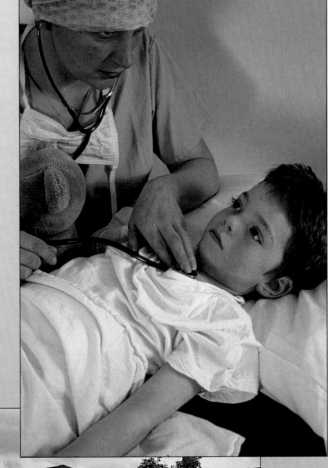

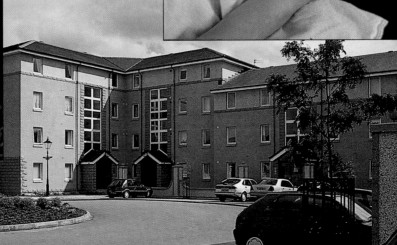

Views about health and wellbeing

What is health? Is it something you're born with, something to do with your body and the way that it works? Or is it more than this? 'Health' is a word that people use all the time but what does it mean? As a student of health and social care you should be clear about what the term can mean. The first part of this unit is about different ways of thinking about health.

The ideas you have about health are those that other people in your society and culture use and have probably taught you. We tend to take these ideas for granted, and sometimes assume that there is only one way of thinking about health. This isn't so. There are many different views about what health means. Chinese or Indian cultures, for example, adopt very different approaches to health and the causes of ill-health from the medical approach typically used in Western societies such as the United Kingdom.

Western ideas about health

For many people living in European and American (Western) societies, being 'healthy' means the absence of any injuries, diseases or simply feeling 'okay'. This is known as a **negative view of health** because being 'healthy' is based on not being or feeling unwell! An alternative, **positive view of health** that is also used in Western societies involves identifying the qualities and abilities that a person ought to have in order to be healthy. For example, being physically fit, the correct weight and feeling happy might be seen as evidence that a person is healthy.

Health seems like a simple idea but it's quite hard to work out what it involves. It's not a fixed quality in a person that can easily be seen or measured. If it was, we could say something like 'all people who are the correct weight for their height are healthy'. However, some of these people might be physically unfit and wouldn't be able to run a mile if they tried. Or they might have illnesses or diseases affecting their physical or mental health.

When you're thinking about health and whether a person is healthy, it's important to take their age and life stage into account. Being able to walk ten miles may be a sign of good **physical health** (or fitness at least) in an 18-year-old, but it isn't something you would expect a 90-year-old person to do even if they were very healthy for their age. Or would you?

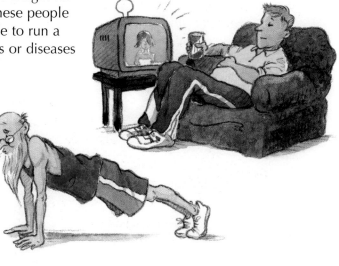

▼ A person can be healthy (or unhealthy) at any age

I'd think that a 90-year old who could walk a mile without help was physically very healthy (or fit) for their age! The last part, 'for their age', is the important point. The way you think about health should take into account a person's age-related needs and abilities. So, we could say that a physically active 90-year old man might be just as physically healthy, considering his age, as his 18-year-old great grandson.

We've said that health isn't just about a fixed or measurable quality, such as physical fitness or weight. So, what else might it involve? People using a **holistic approach** to health say we should take other aspects of a person's life into account when we're looking at their health. They argue that we need to think about the 'whole person' and should look at:

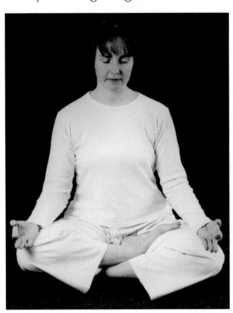

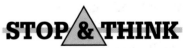
▼ Practising yoga and meditation are ways of helping you to become healthy as a whole person

- physical (bodily) health
- **intellectual** (thinking and learning) wellbeing
- social (relationship) **wellbeing**
- emotional (feelings) **wellbeing**

You may have noticed that the word 'wellbeing' has crept into the discussion about what it means to be healthy. But what does wellbeing involve? How is it different from health?

Wellbeing is used in Western societies to refer to the way people feel about themselves. If people feel 'good' (positive) about themselves and are happy with life, they will have a high level of wellbeing, and vice versa. As individuals, we are the best judges of our personal sense of wellbeing.

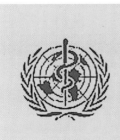

The World Health Organisation takes a **positive** and a **holistic** view when it defines health as:

'a state of complete physical, mental and social wellbeing, not merely the absence of disease or infirmity'

(WHO, 1946).

STOP & THINK

How do you judge your own sense of wellbeing? Have a go at judging this now.

Quick Questions

1 Name three ways of defining health.

2 Explain why a person who is physically fit and the correct weight for their height might not be healthy.

3 What does the term 'emotional wellbeing' refer to?

Ideas about ill-health

If you're not healthy, what are you? Unhealthy, perhaps! There are lots of different ways of describing the absence or lack of health.

In Western societies, health professionals use several different terms to describe a person's lack of health. For example, the terms disease, illness and ill health are commonly used to describe an unhealthy state. What do they mean?

Disease is a term used by doctors and other health care workers to refer to a physical change in the body's correct structure or way of working. Health professionals use the term disease only when they can measure, see or picture (using X-rays or scans perhaps) some type of abnormality.

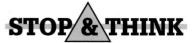

STOP & THINK

Can you think of words people use to describe being or feeling 'unhealthy'? Make a list of ten words. Include words that you use when talking to your friends, family and health workers.

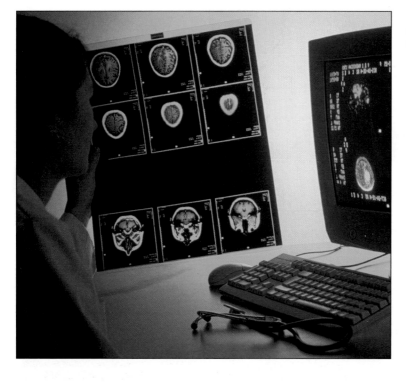

◀ Medical workers use specialist equipment to identify otherwise hidden diseases

How is this different to an illness? A person with an illness may complain that he or she feels unwell and has symptoms, such as aches and pains. However, these symptoms can't always be directly seen or observed by others. This doesn't mean that the person is making up their symptoms or that there is nothing wrong with them! It means that they don't feel in good health and that physically, emotionally or mentally they're not at their best. Illnesses are usually seen as less serious and are a more temporary threat to health than diseases. Even so, Western doctors and other health professionals see many people each day who feel ill and want their help to get over their temporary health problems.

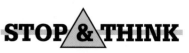

STOP & THINK

Can you think of an example of a disease and an illness? Use the explanation in the text to guide your choices.

People can have a disease (a change in their body) without feeling ill or noticing that anything is wrong. This is one of the reasons for having **screening programmes**. Cervical smears, breast screening after the age of 50, childhood blood tests and chest X-rays are all carried out to identify diseases that in their early stages often don't cause people to feel ill.

Impairment and disability

People may be born with or can develop physical, mental or sensory **impairment**, or damage to part of their body. For example, a person born with Down's Syndrome will have an *intellectual* impairment because the condition affects their ability to develop thinking skills. Similarly, a person who has an accident and loses a leg is said to have a *physical* impairment which will affect their ability to walk unaided, or to do some other physical activities. Does an 'impairment', such as those mentioned, mean that a disabled person is not 'healthy'?

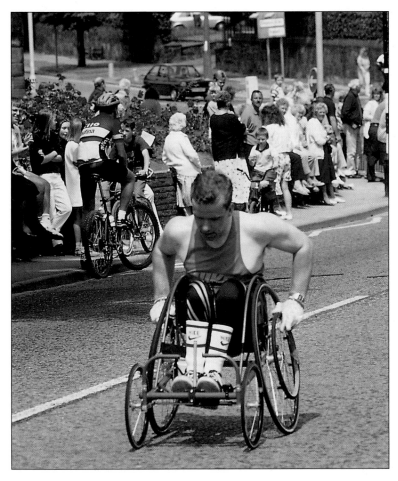

◄ Disabled athletes are often very physically fit

Disabled athletes provide very good evidence that having some form of impairment doesn't necessarily mean that a person will be physically unhealthy or unwell. They prove that people can be 'healthy' despite missing limbs, or not having certain 'taken-for-granted' abilities, such as sight.

Quick Questions

1 Name two ways by which a health professional can tell whether an individual has a disease.

2 Why is it incorrect to assume that a person who has some form of impairment is also unhealthy?

3 Identify an example of a health-screening programme and explain the purpose of screening programmes.

Health in the past

People have thought about health and wellbeing in a variety of different ways for thousands of years. Many of these ideas seem unusual to us by present-day standards. Ideas about health have changed over time, but many present-day thoughts and theories about what it means to be 'healthy' have evolved, or been developed, from these earlier ideas.

People have always thought about health and tried to work out what it involves. Whatever historical period they've lived in, people needed to know how to avoid disease and illness, how to deal with sickness and how to be, and remain, 'healthy'.

It is hard to get evidence from prehistoric times. However, a possible source of evidence about 'health' ideas is found in the skulls discovered by archaeologists and dated as belonging to the period – about 17,000 years ago. Some of these skulls had holes drilled in them. One theory is that prehistoric people did this to release the 'spirit' of a person who had died. However, many of the skulls show evidence that the person survived this operation and was therefore alive when it happened! Was this procedure, known as trepanning, part of the health beliefs and treatment approach of prehistoric people?

More recent evidence from nomadic and non-industrialised societies shows that in the not-too-distant past some cultures based their beliefs about health and the causes of illness on the existence and work of spirits and gods. In some cultures, good and bad spirits were seen to affect everyday life and to cause a person to suffer from illness, or even die, by entering their body. The cure for this was to rid the body of the evil spirit. A religious leader or traditional healer would be called on to banish the spirit from the person and return them to health. These ideas are very different from those of present-day Western societies.

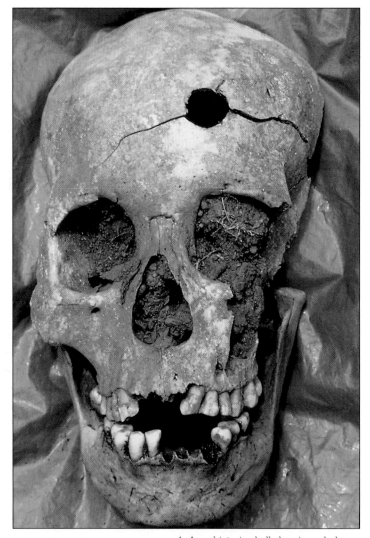

▲ A prehistoric skull showing a hole likely to have been made by a drill

Ideas about health and ill health in the United Kingdom changed significantly with the development of scientific thinking in the eighteenth century. People began to move away from the belief that magic, evil spirits or a disapproving god controlled health and illness. The development of microscopes, knowledge about human anatomy and understanding of body chemistry resulted in the emergence of medical and scientific approaches to health and ways of dealing with ill-health. Based on theories and observations of how the human body works, these ideas about health and ill-health are those that we currently recognise and use as 'true'. Instead of having religious leaders and traditional healers to banish evil spirits, we now have doctors and other health professionals to put our ideas about health into practice.

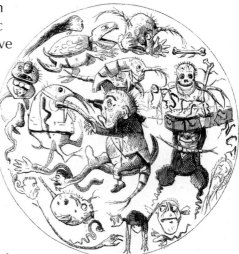

▲ An 1850 Punch cartoon showing 'a drop of London water' and the nasty diseases it contained

Knowledge and understanding about health and wellbeing is always developing. What will people think about the nature and causes of health in 20, 50 or 100 years' time? Will ideas be radically different in 2000 years – as they are now when we look back at earlier ideas? Will people look back and think our current ideas are as unsophisticated and odd as we do when we look at the evil spirit theories?

It's important to remain open minded about health, and the causes and best ways of treating ill-health. Even though they don't fit in with present-day medical views, many of the apparently old and unusual ideas about health from earlier times and different cultures continue to be used in the United Kingdom, and throughout the world. This is often because they work by helping people to get over health problems and by making them feel better. Ongoing research into traditional cures and treatments also shows that the ideas of the past were sometimes based on good sense, and played an important part in improving people's lives at the time. For example, modern scientists are now finding that the plants and herbs used by ancient civilisations as painkillers and sedatives provide very effective forms of 'natural' treatment. In fact, many modern-day medicines are produced from plants and herbs – aspirin, for example, comes from willow bark.

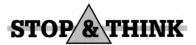

STOP & THINK

Are you superstitious about anything? Think about your superstitions and how they affect the ways that you act or behave. Are any of your superstitious beliefs linked to ideas about health or ill-health?

Health ideas from the past

- Ancient Egyptians used a sand-paste to clean their teeth.

- Aboriginal peoples used a casing of mud and clay to set broken limbs, and clear their camps of human waste and debris to stop their enemies stealing their spirits.

- Aztec Indians used human hair to stitch body wounds.

Quick Questions

1 What is 'trepanning'?

2 Describe a non-medical way of thinking about the causes of ill-health.

3 Explain why we no longer tend to believe that health and illness result from the action of 'evil spirits'.

Health in other cultures

We mentioned earlier that Western ideas about health and wellbeing are different from those of some other cultures. For example, Chinese herbal medicine today is based on ideas about health that are 2000 years old. These ideas result in a different approach to health and ill-health from that used by most people in the United Kingdom.

Chinese herbal medicine deals with both physical and mental health problems. It also provides ways of strengthening a person's recovery power, their immunity and capacity for wellbeing. Chinese herbal medicine is being used increasingly in Western countries and is growing in popularity.

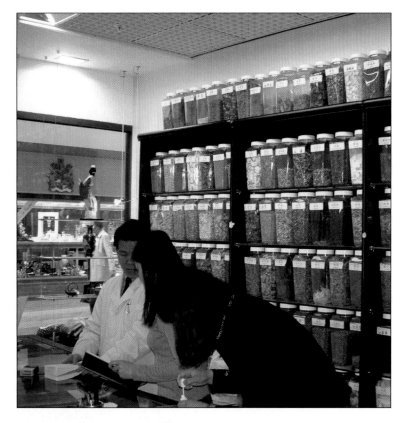

◄ Chinese medicine uses many different herbal substances

Consulting a Chinese herbalist

You've probably been to see a doctor at some point in your life. You'd know what to expect if you went to a GP surgery and made an appointment. The GP would use his or her knowledge of Western medicine and ideas about health and illness to try and diagnose (identify) your health problems. It's less likely that you've been to see a practitioner of Chinese herbal medicine. What do they do? How would they try to diagnose your health problems?

A Chinese herbal medicine practitioner will try to diagnose the 'patterns of disharmony' affecting you. They will be trying to work out whether you have blocked, deficient or disturbed 'energy' (ch'i). Once they discover how your 'energy' is 'blocked', the Chinese herbalist will prescribe a range of herbal medicines and give you advice on how to restore your normal 'energy' balance.

How is diagnosis carried out?

You visit a Chinese herbalist with a 'complaint'. The herbalist asks you what the complaint is, where it is, whether it comes and goes, how intense it is, what makes it better or worse (food, activity, time of day, for example), and what you have done about it. The herbalist collects this information to identify your 'patterns of dysfunction'. The herbalist will also feel your pulse and look closely at your tongue to look for signs of 'imbalance'. According to the Chinese system, healthy people need to achieve a mind–spirit balance, an energy balance, a blood balance and a body fluids balance. The herbal medicines that you will be prescribed are said to strengthen your organs or to 'clear' from your body the unhealthy factors that are preventing balance and blocking energy flows.

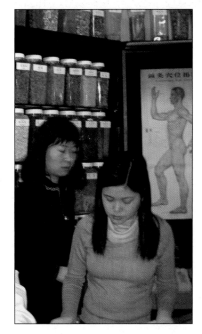

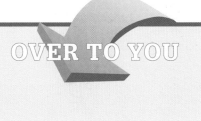

OVER TO YOU

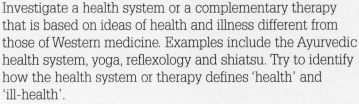

Investigate a health system or a complementary therapy that is based on ideas of health and illness different from those of Western medicine. Examples include the Ayurvedic health system, yoga, reflexology and shiatsu. Try to identify how the health system or therapy defines 'health' and 'ill-health'.

Quick Questions

1 Name two physical features that a Chinese medical herbalist would look closely at when assessing a person's health problems.

2 What, according to Chinese herbal medicine, happens to cause a person to be unwell?

3 Describe the purpose of the herbal medicines which are prescribed by Chinese herbalists.

Who is healthy?

The six people described below have different lifestyles, attitudes, values and needs. In some ways they may be 'healthy', in other ways they may not be. Read through each case study and then answer the Quick Questions at the end.

Lois, age 30, has a job as a stockbroker. She buys and sells shares and must reach certain targets each week. She works out in the company gym each morning and then works very hard from 7.30 a.m. to 7.30 p.m. five days a week. She admits to feeling stressed most of the time. Before going home, she usually goes for a few drinks with her colleagues to wind down. She has made a lot of money but says that she has little time for other things.

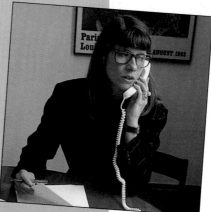

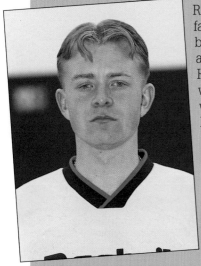

Richie is a 27-year-old packer in a factory. He says his job is very boring. His life really revolves around sport and fitness training. He goes to a gym five nights a week to do weight training. Before work each day, he jogs or swims. He cycles everywhere he goes. Richie is very concerned about his diet and his physical appearance. He thinks about exercise even when he isn't doing it. He always wants to do more to improve his body. He has recently started taking anabolic steroids to help him build up his physique.

Amira describes herself as 'just a housewife'. She is 23 and has two children under five. She lives on income support, but occasionally gets help from her mother who lives a few miles away. She says that the children take up most of her time so she doesn't go out very often. Her favourite pastime is television. After the children are in bed she likes to watch soap operas and quiz shows. She always has a box of chocolates, some crisps and a few cans of lemonade while she watches TV.

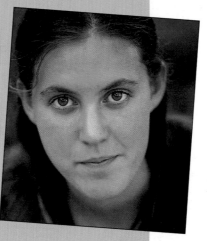

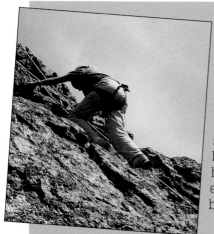

Linda is a 19-year-old student of geology. In her first year at university, she joined a rock climbing group and went on most of their climbing trips. She recently went on a trip to Snowdonia. This time, she says, she 'just lost her nerve'. She got stuck on a cliff face and had to be taken off by rescue helicopter. She's been feeling 'on edge' ever since and has fallen behind in her studies this term.

Alex, age 47, gave up his job as a business studies lecturer two years ago to live in France and write books. He used to spend a great deal of time out of doors, cycling around the countryside. Last year he damaged his ankle in a fall and can no longer ride very far. Although he's made a few friends, he rarely has enough money to go out. Last winter he felt lonely. He caught pneumonia because he couldn't afford to heat his house. He's now working as a tourist guide to make money until he gets a book published.

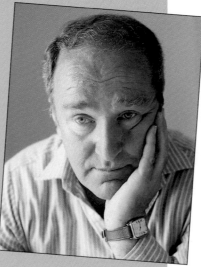

Gary is a 55-year-old nurse working on a hospital medical ward. He works seven days a week, sometimes doing two seven-hour shifts (one in the morning, the other in the afternoon) and finishing at 9.30 p.m. He's very concerned about hygiene and always uses disposable gloves at work. Gary washes his hands several times during the day. He carries an extra suit of clothing to change into between shifts. He's worried he might contract a serious disease and insists that his house is cleaned every day, with a fresh set of bed linen put on every other day. His spare time is spent sleeping.

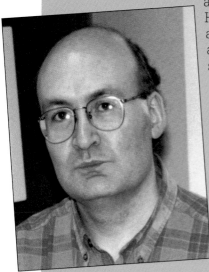

Quick Questions

1 In what way is each person healthy or unhealthy? Make notes of your ideas. You might want to give each person a score (10 = extremely healthy, 1 = extremely unhealthy) for physical, emotional, social and intellectual health.

2 Compare and discuss your ideas and scores with other people in the class.

3 What sort of approach to health are you using in making your decision about each person? (Hint: is your approach to health positive, negative or some other approach?)

Build Your Learning

LEARNING POINTS

The following are the main points that you should have learnt from the previous 10 pages.

- There are number of different ways of thinking about 'health' and 'wellbeing'.
- Western societies use both positive and negative definitions of health and wellbeing.
- Ideas about health and wellbeing vary between different cultures and change over time.

REVISION QUESTIONS

If you're confident that you understand the learning points and the key terms, try answering the revision questions below:

1 What is the difference between:

a) health and wellbeing?

b) a negative and a positive view of health?

c) illness and disease?

d) intellectual wellbeing and social wellbeing?

2 Explain what is meant by a holistic approach to health and wellbeing.

3 Describe, using examples, how ideas about 'health' can vary over time and between different cultures.

The key question that you should be able to answer if you've understood the previous section is:

4 'What is health and wellbeing?' Write an answer to this in your own words.

KEY TERMS

You should know what the following terms mean:

- Health (page 86)
- Negative view of health (page 86)
- Positive view of health (page 86)
- Physical health (page 86)
- Wellbeing (page 87)
- Intellectual wellbeing (page 87)
- Social wellbeing (page 87)
- Emotional wellbeing (page 87)
- Holistic approach (page 87)
- Disease (page 88)
- Illness (page 88)
- Screening programmes (page 89)
- Impairment (page 89)
- Trepanning (page 90)
- Chinese herbal medicine (page 92)

If you're not sure or want to check your understanding, turn to the page number listed in the brackets.

INVESTIGATION IDEAS

1 Carry out a survey of your family and friends to find out how they think about 'health'. You'll need to prepare some questions to ask them or a questionnaire for them to complete. Summarise your results by comparing what different people say about the various approaches to 'health' we've looked at.

2 Do some local research to find complementary health practitioners. Try to get information about the services that these practitioners offer, and the ways in which they think about 'health'.

3 Use the library or the internet to get more information about non-western approaches to health, such as the Ayurvedic health system or Chinese medicine.

Would you like to be healthy? Most people would answer 'yes' to this question. Research has shown that people say being healthy is just as likely to make them feel happy as winning lots of money. Which would you prefer to have – good health or lots of money? You'd have to be very lucky to win lots of money. Being healthy is a bit easier to achieve. So, what sorts of things would help you to be healthy? What are the secrets of health and happiness? You could introduce the following measures and try to make them part of your life.

- Eat *nutritious food* and have a *balanced diet*.
- Take regular *exercise*.
- Get enough *rest* and *sleep*.
- Form *supportive relationships* with others.
- Have *enough money*.
- Obtain and enjoy *work, education* and *leisure activities*.
- Use *available health monitoring* and *illness prevention services*.
- Stay safe and *avoid accidents*.

Now you know at least part of the secret of being healthy and happy! Your chances of being healthy will be a lot higher if you understand how and why each of these factors has a positive effect on health.

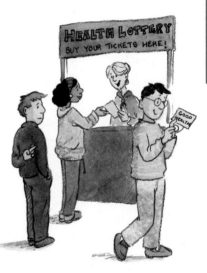

▲ Would winning lots of money make a difference to your health or wellbeing?

Food and health

Food plays a very important role in health. The food we eat should be nutritious if it is going to be beneficial to our physical health. This means it should contain a variety of nutrients. **Nutrients** are naturally occurring chemical substances found in the food we eat.

There are five basic nutrients which help the body in different ways:

- **Carbohydrates** and **fats** provide the body with energy.
- **Proteins** provide the chemical substances needed to build and repair body cells and tissues.
- **Vitamins** help to regulate the chemical reactions that continuously take place in our bodies.
- **Minerals** are needed for control of body functions and to build and repair certain tissues.

As well as eating food that contains a balance of these five nutrients, we also need to consume **fibre** and **water**. Although these are not counted as nutrients they are vital for physical health.

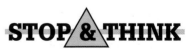

STOP & THINK

Do you know which foods contain the different nutrients? Identify at least two sources of each nutrient in the food you eat regularly.

A healthy intake of food, also known as a **balanced diet**, contains suitable amounts of each of the five basic nutrients. The amount and types of foods that are healthy for a person to eat, varies for each individual. The factors that affect how much and what types of food we need include:

- age
- gender
- body size
- height
- weight
- the environment (for example, whether you live in a cold or a warm country)
- the amount of physical activity you do in your daily life.

Nutrition is very important in the early years of life. Babies and infants need the right types of food to help them grow and develop normally, and to prevent them from developing certain illnesses. Children and adolescents also need the right types of food to promote their physical growth and to provide 'fuel' or energy for their high level of physical activity.

People who have special diets, for example vegetarians and vegans, leave out or include specific food groups to meet their personal values. **Vegetarians** don't eat meat or fish but they can still get all the nutrients they need. They can get proteins from cereals, beans, eggs and cheese. **Vegans**, who eat no animal products at all, can get all their essential nutrients provided their food intake is varied. For example, they can get protein from nuts and pulses.

Family member	Day	Breakfast
Tom age 40	Saturday	Boiled egg, toast, coffee
	Sunday	Fried egg, bacon, toast, coffee
Laura age 30	Saturday	Boiled egg, toast, tea
	Sunday	Toast, marmalade, orange juice, tea
Rachel age 8	Saturday	Cornflakes, orange juice
	Sunday	Fried egg, toast, orange juice
Danny age 3	Saturday	Ready breakfast cereal, milk
	Sunday	Toast, savoury spread, milk
Audrey age 73	Saturday	Grapefruit, crispbread, marmalade, tea
	Sunday	Boiled egg, toast, tea

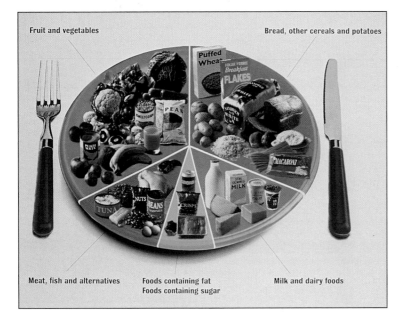

Fruit and vegetables

Bread, other cereals and potatoes

Meat, fish and alternatives

Foods containing fat
Foods containing sugar

Milk and dairy foods

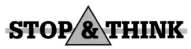

STOP & THINK

Why do you think that a woman might need to adjust her diet when she is pregnant, and when she reaches old age?

OVER TO YOU

Lunch	Snacks	Dinner
Ham roll, crisps,	Doughnut, coffee	Pizza, salad, baked beans, baked potatoes, beer, chocolate cake
Roast chicken, roast potatoes, peas, carrots, tinned fruit, ice cream, white wine	Chocolate bar, coffee	Cheese and pickle sandwich, fruit cake, tea
Crispbread, cottage cheese, herb tea,	Apple, diet coke	Pizza, salad, diet coke, orange, coffee
Roast chicken, peas, carrots, ice cream, wine, coffee	Banana, diet coke	Fruit cake, tea
Ham roll, crisps, blackcurrant squash	Chocolate bar, cola drink	Pizza, salad, baked potato, blackcurrant squash, chocolate cake
Roast chicken, roast potatoes, carrots, ice cream, wafers, grape juice	Cheese sandwich,	Chocolate milkshake; sponge cake
Tuna sandwich, apple, orange juice	Chocolate bar, milk	Pizza, salad, blackcurrant squash, chocolate cake
Roast chicken, roast potato, peas, ice cream, wafers, grape juice	Chocolate milkshake	Fruit yoghurt, sponge cake, blackcurrant squash
Roll, cottage cheese, tomato, herb tea	Apple	Pizza, salad, chocolate cake, tea
Roast chicken, roast potato, peas, carrots, tinned fruit, ice cream, wine, coffee	Nothing	Tuna sandwich, fruit cake, tea

This is a diet record sheet showing the weekend food consumption for members of the James family (who we'll meet in Unit 3). Use the diet sheet to answer these questions:

1 Indicate which nutrients can be found in the foods eaten by the family.

2 Identify the effect of each nutrient on the body.

3 How nutritional is this family's diet?

4 Do you think that individual family members are getting a balanced diet?

5 Are there any deficiencies or excesses in their nutritional intakes?

Using examples from the record sheet, write a paragraph explaining your views on the last three questions. What advice would you give to the parents of Danny and Rachel about the type of diet needed to promote healthy growth and development in children?

Quick Questions

1 Name the five basic nutrients that are part of a balanced diet.
2 Describe the factors that affect how much food a person should eat.
3 Explain why a varied and balanced diet is especially important for babies and children.

Exercise

Do you like doing exercise? Some people really enjoy sports, going to the gym or doing exercise classes. You might be one of them. Or you might be one of the large number of people who don't do enough exercise. Unfortunately exercise isn't as popular as eating food and is one of the things in our top health tips list that many people struggle with. But it's still important, and is very good for your physical health.

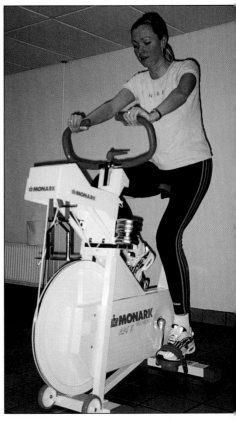

▲ Exercise is good for both physical and mental health

Benefits of exercise

Exercise…

…keeps the heart healthy

…improves circulation

…helps muscles, joints and bones to remain strong

…improves stamina

…reduces blood pressure

…increases self-esteem and self-confidence

…helps to control and maintain weight

…makes you feel more energetic

…is a good way of socialising

…helps the body to stay supple and mobile

Exercise has a positive effect on both physical and mental health. But it's important not to do too much. People should find a balance between physical activity and rest in order to maintain good physical health and a sense of wellbeing.

So, what kinds of exercise should you do? The type and level of exercise that an individual can do safely depends on their age, gender and health status. For example, moderate exercise can be safely undertaken by older and less physically mobile people, including women in the later stages of pregnancy and people with physical disabilities. Younger people who are physically fit can safely undertake more vigorous exercise.

Lack of physical exercise can lead to ill health and disease. For example, lack of exercise is linked to an increased risk of diseases such as coronary heart disease, stroke, obesity (being excessively overweight) and osteoporosis (brittle bones). Obesity is now a major health problem in the United Kingdom and is closely linked to people overeating and not exercising. There are many reasons why people don't take more exercise. These include not having enough time, not liking sport and being frightened of injuries.

Rest and sleep

Do you get enough rest and sleep? How much sleep do you need to be healthy? If you want to be healthy you've got to take rest and sleep seriously. Not everyone does. Some people work too much and spend their life feeling tired. This isn't healthy.

People should rest every day to maintain their health and wellbeing. The amount of sleep a person needs varies according to their age. Babies, young children, older people and pregnant women tend to need a period of rest (lack of exertion) during the day.

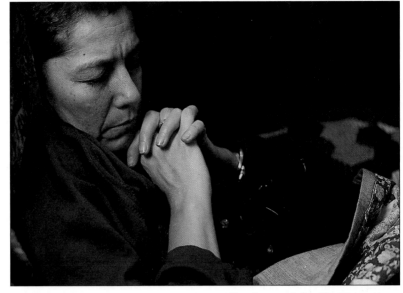

▲ Rest is part of a healthy life

Most healthy adults and older children need to rest only at the end of their active day. Even so, people need varying amounts of sleep depending on their life stage and physical needs. For example, a four-year-old child sleeps an average of ten to fourteen hours a day whilst a ten-year-old needs about nine to twelve hours. Most adults sleep from seven to eight and a half hours every night. Others require as few as four or five hours or as many as ten hours each night. Most people find that they need slightly less sleep as they grow older. A person who slept eight hours a night when they were thirty years old may need only six or seven hours when they are sixty years old.

What happens if you don't get enough rest and sleep? People who are deprived of sleep lose energy and become irritable. After two days without sleep, concentration becomes difficult. Other negative, and potentially dangerous, effects of sleep loss include:

- mistakes in routine tasks
- slips of attention
- dozing off for periods of a few seconds or more
- falling asleep completely
- difficulty seeing and hearing clearly
- confusion.

Lack of sleep can be very dangerous. For example, many car accidents are caused by people falling asleep while driving and losing control of their vehicle.

Quick Questions

1 Name one physical, one social and one emotional benefit of regular exercise.

2 Describe the effects of having insufficient rest and sleep.

3 Explain why having a balance between activity and rest is important for a healthy lifestyle.

The role of supportive relationships

Have you got good friends and relatives who you care about? Hopefully you will be able to think of a variety of people who are emotionally close to you. These people are good for your health and wellbeing. You may have disagreements and fall out with family members and close friends from time to time, but you shouldn't underestimate the important effect they have on your emotional wellbeing.

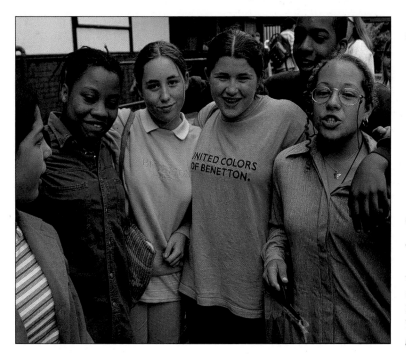

◄ Friendships are very important for our emotional wellbeing

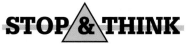

Who do you have close, supportive relationships with? Try and identify how each of your supportive relationships contributes to your sense of wellbeing.

Relationships with friends and relatives are supportive when the people involved feel emotionally close, cared for and able to trust each other. We need supportive relationships in each life stage to experience wellbeing, and to support our social and emotional development.

Babies and children generally have their closest relationship with their parents or main carers. Babies need to develop close attachments with an adult carer so that they can develop emotionally and experience a secure relationship. A supportive relationship with parents or a carer allows a growing child to develop their self-concept and self-esteem.

▼ Good parent-child relationships are essential for emotional development

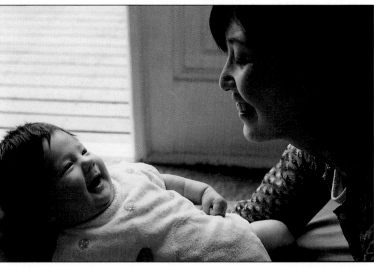

Psychologists believe that our first relationship provides a blueprint for all future relationships. If it is supportive, it's more likely that we'll develop healthy relationships later in life.

Close friendships with other children become more important during childhood. Children tend to select one or two others as close friends and gain a lot of social and emotional support in this way. Not having friends can lead to a child feeling 'left out' and having low self-esteem.

During adolescence, close supportive relationships with friends and parents provide people with a 'safe place' when they feel stressed and under pressure. These supportive relationships help to boost self-esteem, a sense of belonging and a sense of feeling valued by others.

During adulthood and old age, supportive relationships with children, partners, friends and other family members are important for self-esteem and emotional wellbeing. Lack of supportive relationships can result in a person feeling isolated, lonely and depressed. Researchers have shown that people who lack close, supportive relationships are much more likely to experience depression.

STOP & THINK

How do you think parents can develop supportive relationships with their children? Suggest ways in which parents can build up an emotionally close relationship with their children.

CASE STUDY

Robbie is one year old. Monica, his mum, is 22 years old and a lone parent. She has recently found out that she has to go in to hospital for an eye operation. Monica is upset and feels frightened about how this might turn out. Her worst fear is that something will go wrong and she won't able to care for Robbie afterwards. She's also upset about the prospect of being separated from Robbie for a week while she's in hospital.

- How might Robbie react if he feels insecure and unsupported when Monica is admitted to hospital?

- Who would you seek support from if you were in Monica's situation?

- What kinds of support do you think Monica needs at the moment?

- What do you think the care staff at the hospital could do to build a supportive relationship with Monica while she's a patient there?

Quick Questions

1 Identify one quality or characteristic of a supportive relationship.

2 Who do babies and young children usually have supportive relationships with?

3 Explain why supportive relationships are thought to be important for health and wellbeing.

Is money linked to health and wellbeing?

Money is an **economic factor** linked to health and wellbeing. How much money would you need to be healthy? Is there an answer to this or is it a silly question? Money is not directly linked to health – having more money doesn't make a person healthier. Despite this, money does play a very important part in our health and wellbeing.

The amount of money that people earn affects their lifestyle and their opportunities. People need enough money (adequate finance) to afford the basic necessities of life, such as food, housing and clothing, which directly affect physical health. People with more money generally have better housing and may eat better quality food. In this way money does affect basic physical health.

People who have a good income are less likely to worry about being able to cope with everyday life. They don't experience the same stress as people who are worried about paying their rent or feeding their children, for example. Having a good income allows people to buy luxuries such as holidays, cars, electrical goods and other desirable things. It also has a positive effect on self-esteem as money is highly valued in Western societies. People with lots of money are typically seen in a positive way. Being rich and successful is seen as desirable.

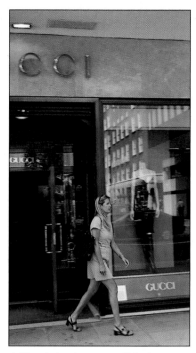

▲ How is having money linked to health?

OVER TO YOU

When we say that people need 'enough money', what do we mean? 'Enough' for what? For the essentials – the basic necessities of life – usually.

1 From the list opposite identify what you think are the basic necessities of life by making two lists:
   a) what you think are basic necessities
   b) what you think are not essentials.

2 How much money would a person need (each week, month or year) to afford your list of basic necessities?

heating ☐   an indoor toilet ☐   satellite TV ☐

a damp-free home ☐   a washing machine ☐

a bath or shower ☐   a foreign holiday ☐

beds for everyone ☐   a mobile 'phone ☐

money for public transport ☐   toys for children ☐

a warm waterproof coat ☐   a refrigerator ☐

access to a personal computer ☐   carpets ☐

three meals a day ☐   a bedroom for each child ☐

two pairs of all-weather shoes ☐

party celebrations ☐   a roastdinner once a week ☐

Work, education and leisure

How do work, education and leisure help people to experience good health and wellbeing? It's useful to use a holistic approach when thinking about this.

The physical activity and exertion involved affect a person's fitness. For example, firemen, builders and fitness instructors do lots of physical exercise in the course of their daily work. Other jobs, such as nursing and shop work, may not be as physically strenuous but still involve a lot of physical activity. Work that is mentally demanding can stimulate a person's intellectual (thinking) development, and be a big motivating factor in their life. Work can also be an important source of self-esteem and status. Health and social care workers, for example, often choose this type of work because they want to be useful and make a difference to peoples' lives. In this way, work has a positive effect on their emotional wellbeing.

How can education affect health and wellbeing in a positive way? The answer is very similar to the effects of work on wellbeing. A person's educational achievements affect their outlook on life, their sense of emotional wellbeing and their self-esteem. For example, people feel proud of passing exams and gaining qualifications, and upset about failing them. Education has a very important effect on a person's intellectual development, and is equally important in the social development of children and young people. Making friends, learning how to communicate and understanding other people are important skills that we learn during our time at school.

Even though work can be good for health and wellbeing, too much can lead to a person feeling stressed and tired.

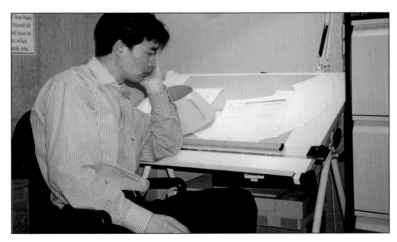

If you want to live a healthy life, it's important to have a balance in your life between work and non-work time. Leisure time, including having hobbies, enjoying a social life and simply relaxing, is part of a healthy life.

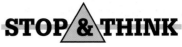

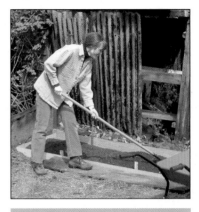

How might work be good for a person's physical health?

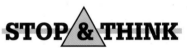

What types of leisure and recreational activities are part of your school/life balance? How do these activities contribute to your health and wellbeing?

Quick Questions

1 Name one positive effect that work can have on a person's health or wellbeing.

2 Which area of health and wellbeing is affected when a person succeeds in their exams?

3 Explain why an active social life and having hobbies can be good for wellbeing.

Health monitoring and illness prevention

The general health of the United Kingdom population is much better now than it was at the beginning of the twentieth century. The evidence for this can be seen in the much higher proportion of children who survive early childhood and the fact that both men and women can now expect to live much longer lives.

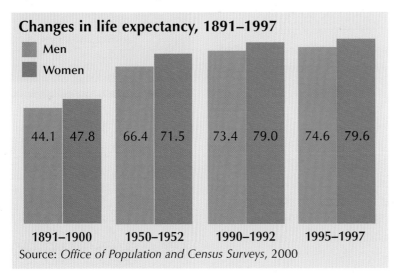

Changes in life expectancy, 1891–1997

■ Men
■ Women

1891–1900		1950–1952		1990–1992		1995–1997	
44.1	47.8	66.4	71.5	73.4	79.0	74.6	79.6

Source: *Office of Population and Census Surveys*, 2000

There are many reasons for the improvements in health that occurred during the twentieth century. One factor was the introduction and use of health monitoring strategies and illness prevention services.

Do you use all the health services that are available to you? When was the last time you had a health check up? Do you check aspects of your own health? Using health monitoring and illness prevention services, and assessing your own health regularly, are all good ways of achieving and maintaining good physical health and wellbeing.

Many of the health services now available are not there to treat health problems, such as diseases and illnesses. Instead, they aim to prevent people from developing problems or from getting ill in the first place. They do this through various health monitoring and illness prevention methods.

Health monitoring can be carried out both by health professionals, through regular check ups and screening programmes, and also by people who've learnt simple self-monitoring techniques, such as breast self-examination. Checking your weight, looking after your skin and hair and having regular dental check ups and eye tests are all ways of monitoring personal health.

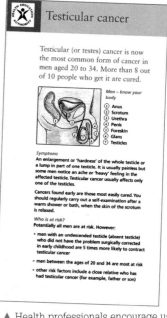

Testicular cancer

Testicular (or testes) cancer is now the most common form of cancer in men aged 20 to 34. More than 8 out of 10 people who get it are cured.

Men – know your body
① Anus
② Scrotum
③ Urethra
④ Penis
⑤ Foreskin
⑥ Glans
⑦ Testicles

Symptoms
An enlargement or 'hardness' of the whole testicle or a lump in part of one testicle. It is usually painless but some men notice an ache or 'heavy' feeling in the affected testicle. Testicular cancer usually affects only one of the testicles.

Cancers found early are those most easily cured. You should regularly carry out a self-examination after a warm shower or bath, when the skin of the scrotum is relaxed.

Who is at risk?
Potentially all men are at risk. However:

• men with an undescended testicle (absent testicle) who did not have the problem surgically corrected in early childhood are 5 times more likely to contract testicular cancer

• men between the ages of 20 and 34 are most at risk

• other risk factors include a close relative who has had testicular cancer (for example, father or son)

▲ Health professionals encourage us to help monitor our own health

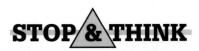

STOP & THINK

Can you think of any health monitoring services designed for babies or children? Make a list of the services available in your area.

Health professionals provide a range of services designed to prevent people from becoming ill and to promote a healthy lifestyle. Taking the advice they offer and using their services can help you to enjoy good health and wellbeing. Services are usually provided for particular client groups, or to deal with particular health problems.

For example, illness prevention services include:

- **Immunisations** against childhood illnesses such as chickenpox and measles; against viruses, such as influenza (flu), that affect many older people; and against tropical diseases, such as malaria, that can affect overseas travellers visiting areas where the virus is prevalent.

- **Advice and information services** to help people change their unhealthy behaviour and live healthier lives. GPs, for example, provide advice about stopping smoking and ways of losing weight.

- **Classes** where health workers teach people ways of improving their health. For example, relaxation and yoga for people who are stressed, or opportunities for people to meet and talk about their problems.

So, health and wellbeing can be improved by using preventative health services, by adjusting your lifestyle and by monitoring your physical health. People who use health monitoring and illness prevention services take an active, positive approach to being healthy and feeling good.

Quick Questions

1 Name two methods used by health professionals to prevent ill-health.

2 Describe one way that a person can monitor their physical health.

3 Explain what an immunisation involves.

CASE STUDY

Joanne is 30 years old. She's been trying to get pregnant since marrying Ray 18 months ago. When she made an appointment with her GP (family doctor), Joanne was hoping that there would be a quick and simple solution to the problem. The GP said he would need to carry out a range of health checks to find out about her health behaviour and life style before he could suggest any solutions. At the end of the consultation, Joanne was encouraged to lose some weight, enrol in relaxation classes at the surgery and improve her diet. The GP said that Joanne should monitor her own health for three months to see if the changes she made had any effect. He told her that being in good physical health would help her to conceive.

- What aspects of Joanne's health would you expect the GP check?

- How could Joanne monitor her own health over the next few months?

- What health monitoring or screening services are available to young women like Joanne?

Avoiding hazards and staying safe

The final advice for achieving health and wellbeing is to stay safe. Accidents are responsible for around 10,000 deaths each year in England. Most people who die as the result of an accident are under the age of 35. Accidents are the most common cause of death in people under the age of 30, and also result in a large amount of serious injury and disability. If you want to be healthy, accidents are best avoided.

Statistics also show that young people are more likely to experience violent crime or attack than other sections of the population. But, how do you avoid being the victim of an accident or a potential attacker? Life can never be completely risk free but there are plenty of ways of reducing the risks and avoiding the hazards that are part of modern life.

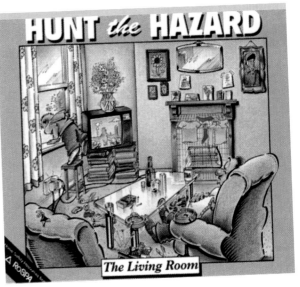

▲ The Royal Society for the Prevention of Accidents (RoSPA) produces posters to help young people identify the many common hazards in our everyday environment

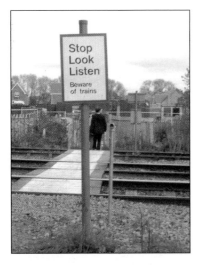

Accident statistics for employed people 1999–2000

Severity of injury	Number of injuries	Injury rate*
Fatal	162	0.7
Non-fatal major	28, 652	116.6
Over-3-day (minor)	135,381	550.6
All injuries	164,195	668.2

*per 100,000 employed
Source: *HSE: Health and social care statistics* 2000–01

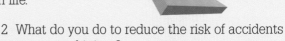

OVER TO YOU

Think about the risks and hazards in your own life.

1 What do you think are the potential hazards in your everyday environment? Think about your journey to school, the environment where you spend your social time and your home environment. Make a list of the main hazards to your health and safety

2 What do you do to reduce the risk of accidents or personal injury?

3 Are there any situations, or places, you avoid because you think the risk of an accident or attack is too high? Describe the situation and suggest ways in which the risks could be reduced or prevented.

If you want to stay safe and healthy, assessment of your own and other people's health and safety should be a part of your everyday life. This doesn't mean you should hibernate and try to live a risk-free life, but that you should be alert to potential hazards and dangers in everyday situations. **Risk assessment** is the procedure you go through when you question whether what you're about to do will be safe. For example, is it a good idea to accept a lift in a car if the driver has been drinking in the pub all night? What might the dangers be? Should you fill your room with candles and burn them for the nice smell because it helps you get to sleep? What might the dangers be? Shouldn't you make sure that somebody walks home with you or picks you up if you're out late at night? You probably know by now what the risks and dangers are of not taking these personal safety precautions. Avoiding accidents and staying safe is achieved through everyday risk assessment, by adjusting your behaviour and by ensuring that other people behave safely whether at home, at work or when you're out enjoying yourself.

Avoiding children having accidents in the home:

- Identify sources of potential danger, such as loose stair carpets and faulty electrical items, and correct them.
- Make sure that dangerous items such as knives, and small objects that can be swallowed, are not left where small children can reach them.
- Lock away medicines and poisonous substances, such as bleach and other cleaning agents, that can be accidentally swallowed.
- Ensure that babies and infants are never left unsupervised.
- Ensure that plastic bags, which present a danger of suffocation, are kept out of children's reach.
- Store all inflammable items, such as matches, lighters, petrol and methylated spirits, out of children's reach.
- Install safety gates to prevent infants from falling downstairs or entering unsafe areas, such as a kitchen.
- Use fireguards on all open fires (including electrical fires).

Quick Questions

1 Approximately how many people are killed through accidents each year?

2 Members of which age group are most likely to experience injury or die as a result of an accident?

3 Explain what the term 'risk assessment' means.

Build Your Learning

LEARNING POINTS

The following are the main points that you should have learnt from the previous 13 pages.

- Health and wellbeing are positively affected by a number of factors.
- An individual can control many of the factors affecting health and wellbeing, such as diet, exercise and health monitoring.
- People can improve their health and wellbeing by making positive, healthy lifestyle choices, and by taking personal responsibility for their health behaviour.

REVISION QUESTIONS

If you're confident that you understand the learning points and the key terms, try answering the revision questions below:

1 What are the health benefits of:
   a) a balanced diet?
   b) regular exercise?
   c) supportive relationships?
   d) immunisations?

2 Describe the positive effects that enjoyable work and leisure activities can have on a person's health and wellbeing.

3 Explain why regular sleep and rest are essential for a child's health and wellbeing.

The key question that you should be able to answer if you've understood the previous section is:

4 'What factors contribute positively to health and wellbeing throughout the life span?' Write an answer in your own words.

KEY TERMS

You should know what the following terms mean:

- Nutrients (page 97)
- Carbohydrates (page 97)
- Fats (page 97)
- Proteins (page 97)
- Vitamins (page 97)
- Fibre (page 97)
- Balanced diet (page 98)
- Vegans (page 98)
- Vegetarians (page 98)
- Obesity (page 100)
- Osteoporosis (page 100)
- Supportive relationships (page 102)
- Economic factor (page 104)
- Leisure (page 105)
- Health monitoring (page 106)
- Immunisation (page 107)
- Risk assessment (page 109)

If you're not sure or want to check your understanding, turn to the page number listed in the brackets.

INVESTIGATION IDEAS

1 Use the library or the internet to carry out further research into the ways that nutrition and exercise can have a beneficial effect on physical health. Try to find out how nutritious food and regular exercise have a positive biological effect on the human body.

2 Research the range of immunisations provided for babies and children in the United Kingdom. Produce a summary table outlining the name of each immunisation, the child's age when it is given and any effects. You might find it helpful to ask someone, such as a child care worker or a parent of young children, about the names of the different immunisations. Information about the effects can be found in medical dictionaries and websites.

RISKS TO HEALTH

We have considered how physical, social and economic factors can help people to experience positive health and wellbeing. We've looked at ways of being healthy and feeling good. Now we're going to look at the opposite of health and wellbeing. You could call it 'how to be unhealthy and feel terrible'! In other words, we're going to identify and consider factors known to put health and wellbeing at risk. You may already know of several ways to live an unhealthy life! If any of the factors mentioned are a current feature of your life, you'll learn why you should adjust your lifestyle. If they're not, you'll understand why it's a good idea to keep avoiding them.

Our risks to health and wellbeing guide covers the following factors.

- The effect of INHERITED DISEASES and CONDITIONS on health.
- The dangers of smoking CIGARETTES.
- The dangers of DRINKING too much alcohol.
- The health dangers of DRUG MISUSE.
- The damage that too much STRESS can do to health and wellbeing.
- The impact of poor PERSONAL HYGIENE.
- The possible health consequences of UNPROTECTED SEX.
- The effects that UNEMPLOYMENT can have on health and wellbeing.
- The impact of POOR HOUSING on personal health.
- The health effects of ENVIRONMENTAL POLLUTION.

The information in the following pages doesn't tell you what you should and shouldn't do in your life. That's always up to you. However, it's important to be aware of the possible risks to your health and wellbeing posed by the various factors covered. If you're going to be a health or care worker in the future, a knowledge of the main risks to health will enable you to understand better some of the reasons why the people you care for are experiencing problems.

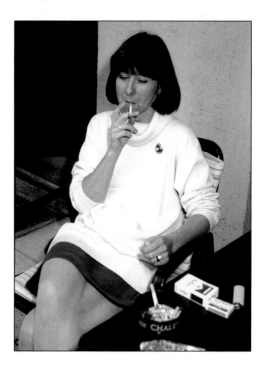

Inherited diseases and conditions

Biologically, you are unique. Your biological uniqueness is a result of the genes that you've inherited from your biological parents. As well as playing a very important role in your physical growth and appearance, the genes you've inherited may also make you vulnerable to some diseases and conditions.

Each human body cell contains two sets of 23 chromosomes – one set from each parent. These chromosomes each contain up to 4,000 different **genes**. The genes we inherit from our parents are the biological 'instructions' or codes that tell our body's cells how to grow. Some people inherit one or more genes that are defective (faulty). These defective genes can result in a person experiencing a disease or condition that has a negative effect on their health and wellbeing. The study of genes, both healthy and defective, is known as **genetics**.

Dominant gene defects

We inherit one set of genes from each of our biological parents. Some of these genes are identical, whilst others differ. For example, we may inherit a blue-eye-colour gene from one parent and a brown-eye-colour gene from the other. Where this happens, one gene will be dominant over the other. (In this situation, the brown-eye-colour gene always wins!)

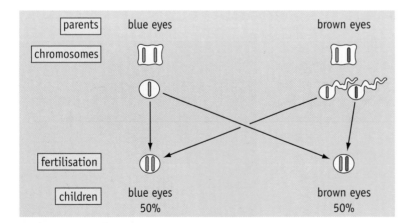

However, if the dominant gene is also a defective gene, the child will inherit the disease or condition for which it provides instruction. For example, people who inherit the defective gene leading to Huntington's disease have a fifty per cent chance of developing the disorder. Huntington's disease is a slowly progressing, fatal brain disorder that results in dementia and uncontrollable movements developing in middle-age. There is now a diagnostic test for people with a family history to assess the risk of them passing the defective gene to their offspring.

Recessive gene defects

A gene that isn't dominant is known as a recessive gene. Normally the genetic information in the recessive gene will be overruled by that in the dominant gene. In the case of eye-colour determination for example, the blue-eye-colour gene is recessive. However, if a person inherits two defective copies of a recessive gene this will have an effect on their health and wellbeing. A person who inherits just one copy will not have the disease or condition but will be a 'carrier' and may pass it on to their children. Cystic fibrosis is a disease inherited as a result of recessive gene defects. Even though about one in every 25 people is a carrier of the faulty recessive gene, only one in every 2,000 children is born with cystic fibrosis.

Chromosomal defects

Some inherited conditions result from a person being born with the wrong number of chromosomes. These include Down's syndrome, Klinefelter's syndrome and Turner's syndrome. All these conditions affect the growth and development of the people who inherit them.

Quick Questions

1 Name one inherited disorder that results from inheriting a recessive gene defect.

2 Describe the effects that Huntington's disease can have on a person's health, wellbeing or development.

3 Explain how a person inherits a disorder as a result of recessive gene defects of their parents.

Cigarette smoking

Do you smoke cigarettes? If not, you probably know people who do. Smoking cigarettes is a prominent part of some people's social life. However, despite being legal and widely available in shops, pubs, clubs and other places of entertainment, cigarettes have got a very bad reputation with health professionals.

Cigarettes, and tobacco smoking of any kind, have no health benefits at all. None. Zero. Nil. Instead, smoking cigarettes directly damages your physical health. This is one of the most important pieces of information that health professionals regularly give out to people. Their advice is always to stop smoking. You should be told this if you smoke cigarettes. People who fail to take note of this warning run a considerable risk of causing themselves long-term health damage and dying, as a direct result of their smoking habit. The health problems associated with smoking tobacco include:

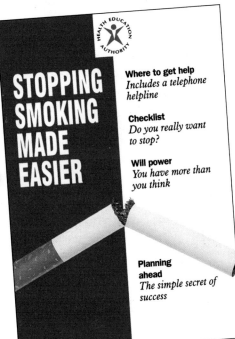

- coronary heart disease
- stroke
- high blood pressure
- bronchitis
- lung cancer
- other cancers, such as cancer of the larynx, kidney and bladder.

Smoking cigarettes is harmful to health because the smoke inhaled and substances circulated deep into the body are harmful. These substances include nicotine, carbon monoxide and tar.

Nicotine is a powerful, fast-acting and addictive drug. Smokers absorb it into their bloodstream and feel an effect in their brains seven to eight minutes later. Some smokers say this is 'calming'. However, the physical effects of smoking also include an increase in heart rate and blood pressure and changes in appetite. Cigarette smoke contains a high concentration of carbon monoxide, a poisonous gas. Carbon monoxide combines more easily than oxygen with haemoglobin (the substance in blood that carries oxygen), so the amount of oxygen carried to a smoker's lungs and tissues is reduced. This reduction in oxygen supply to the body then affects the growth and repair of tissues, and the exchange of essential nutrients.

The carbon monoxide inhaled by a smoker can also affect their heart. The changes in the blood associated with

Year	Men	Women
1949	14.1	6.8
1959	18.4	11.0
1969	18.9	13.7
1979	21.6	16.6
1990	16.8	13.9
2000	14.9	12.7

Source: *General Household Survey 2000* Daily consumption of manufactured cigarettes per smoker, 1949–1998

smoking can cause fat deposits to form on the walls of the arteries. This leads to hardening of the arteries and to circulatory problems, causing smokers to develop coronary heart disease.

Cigarette tar contains many substances known to cause cancer. It damages the cilia, the small hairs lining the lungs that help to protect them from dirt and infection. Because these lung protectors get damaged, smokers are more likely than non-smokers to get throat and chest infections. About 70 per cent of the tar in a cigarette is deposited in the lungs when cigarette smoke is inhaled.

The use of tobacco is now less widespread and less socially acceptable than it was twenty years ago. However, in 1996–7, just under 30 per cent of adults were still smokers and there were over 120,000 smoking-related deaths. Teenage girls are one of the few social groups who are more likely to smoke now than in the past. Tobacco use is therefore still a major cause of preventable disease and early death in the United Kingdom.

Smoking during pregnancy

When women smoke during pregnancy, the ability of the blood to carry oxygen to all parts of the body is reduced. This affects the flow of blood to the placenta, which feeds the fetus. Women who smoke during pregnancy have a greater risk of suffering a miscarriage. Women who smoke tend to give birth to premature and underweight babies who are more prone to upper respiratory tract infections and breathing problems. The risk of cot death among these babies is also increased.

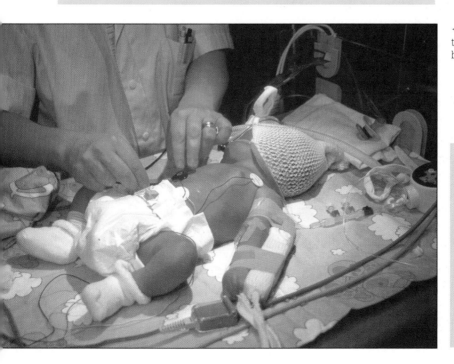

◀ Women who smoke are more likely to have premature and underweight babies

Quick Questions

1 Name three diseases associated with cigarette smoking.

2 Describe the physical effects on the body of inhaling cigarette smoke.

3 Explain what statistics on smoking reveal about the trends of cigarette smoking in the United Kingdom.

Alcohol consumption

Alcohol is a very popular, widely available and accepted part of social life in the United Kingdom. Research shows that 98 per cent of the adult population use alcohol. Many people enjoy a drink and there is usually nothing wrong with that. In small controlled quantities alcoholic drinks can be part of a pleasurable social occasion. In fact, some types of alcoholic drink, such as red wine, have been shown to be good for health.

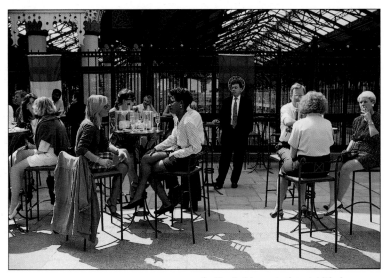

▲ Alcohol is part of social life for many people

The health benefits of alcohol

Studies have shown that people who regularly drink small amounts of alcohol tend to live longer than people who don't drink at all. This is because alcohol protects against the development of coronary heart disease. It also has an effect on the amount of cholesterol, or fat, carried in the bloodstream and, therefore, makes it less likely that the clots which cause heart disease will form. Maximum health advantage can be achieved from drinking between one and two units of alcohol a day. There is no additional overall health benefit to be gained from drinking more than two units of alcohol a day. However, there are possible negative effects from doing so.

When consumed, alcohol is rapidly absorbed into the bloodstream. The amount of alcohol concentrated in the body at any one time depends on how much a person drinks, whether the stomach is empty or full and the height, weight, age and sex of the drinker.

The risks associated with alcohol

Nearly all the alcohol a person drinks has to be burnt up by the liver. The rest is disposed of either in sweat or urine. Your body can get rid of one unit of alcohol in one hour. Smaller than average people, younger or older people and people who are not used to drinking are more easily affected by alcohol and take longer to get it out of their bodies.

Alcohol is a depressant. This means that it reduces certain brain functions and affects judgement, self-control and coordination. This is why alcohol causes fights, domestic violence and accident-related injuries. It has been estimated that up to 40,000 deaths per year could be alcohol related. In 1996, 15 per cent of fatal road accidents resulted from people driving whilst under the influence of alcohol; and it is estimated that 78 per cent of adult drownings involve exessive alcohol consumption.

The health risks associated with alcohol result from consuming it in large quantities, either regularly or in binges. People who frequently drink excess amounts of alcohol have an increased risk of:

- high blood pressure
- coronary heart disease
- liver damage and **cirrhosis** of the liver
- cancer of the mouth and throat
- psychological and emotional problems, including depression
- obesity.

Health professionals recommend safe limits of alcohol consumption. The Department of Health recommends a limit for women of two to three units a day. The recommended limit for men is three to four units a day. One unit of alcohol is the same as one small glass of wine, half a pint of ordinary strength lager, beer or cider, or a 25ml pub measure of spirit. If men and women follow this guide there should be no significant risks to their health. However, if women regularly drink more than three units a day and men drink more than four units a day, the risk to health is increased.

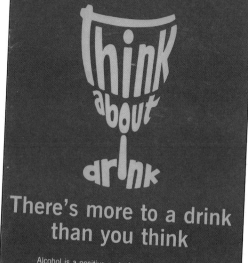

There's more to a drink than you think

Alcohol is a positive part of life for most people. By following the guidelines in this leaflet you can make sure that you can drink alcohol without putting yourself or others at risk.

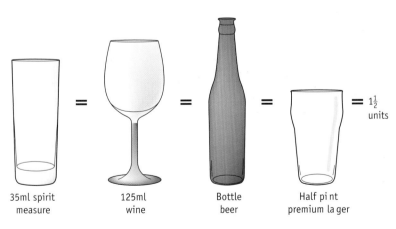

| 35ml spirit measure | 125ml wine | Bottle beer | Half pint premium lager | $1\frac{1}{2}$ units |

You should be aware that these recommended limits are based on 'pub measures'. People who drink at home, or buy alcohol from an off-licence or supermarket to consume elsewhere, usually pour themselves larger measures of wines and spirits or consume stronger beer than that sold in licensed premises (such as pubs, clubs and restaurants).

Quick Questions

1 Name three negative long-term effects that drinking too much alcohol can have on a person's health and wellbeing.

2 What factors should a person take into account when assessing how much it is safe for them to drink?

3 Excessive consumption of alcohol may *indirectly* lead to a person experiencing injury or harm. Explain how alcohol can play a part in people sustaining accidental and non-accidental injuries.

Drug misuse

Drug misuse is very high up the list of ways to harm your health. Damage to health from drug misuse can be sudden and catastrophic (people die) or it can occur over a longer period of time. Either way, drug misuse is something to avoid if you wish to live a long and healthy life.

Drugs are chemical substances that affect the body's chemistry and functioning. Drugs are widely used, and also widely misused, in the United Kingdom. They can be obtained through:

- a doctor's prescription if they are for medical treatment
- over the counter, by purchasing them in a chemist, supermarket or other shop (these drugs include medicines and legal substances such as alcohol and tobacco)
- buying 'street' and medicinal drugs illegally.

For many years, newspapers and television have featured stories and programmes about drug misuse. Drug misuse is now a major cause of health problems and premature death in the United Kingdom. All sections of the population are affected by it, but young people are the most likely to risk their health through drug misuse. There are many complex reasons for this.

Any drug, whether it is legal or illegal, can cause harm if it is misused. For example, whilst medicines are used to treat disease and illness, they can also have physical and psychological side-effects. The doctor who prescribes them will know about these possible effects and will take care to monitor the patient. To limit side effects, the doctor will prescribe only the dose required. People may misuse prescription drugs by taking more than their doctor prescribes, or they may take medicines not prescribed for them. They then run the risk of experiencing harmful and even fatal side-effects.

Percentage of 16 to 24 year olds who have used drugs in the past year, 1998 – England and Wales

	Percentages		
	Male	Female	All
Cannabis	32	22	27
Amphetamines	12	8	10
Ecstasy	6	4	5
Magic mushrooms	5	2	4
LSD	5	2	3
Cocaine	4	3	3
Any drug	36	24	29

Source: *Social Trends 30*, © 2000 HMSO

STOP & THINK

Why do you think some people take illegal drugs? Make a list of possible reasons. Why do other people avoid using them? Make another list of possible reasons.

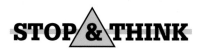

OVER TO YOU

Aspirin and paracetamol are both commonly available drugs that can be obtained by prescription or bought over the counter at a chemist or other shop. But they have harmful side-effects and can be fatal if misused. Find out what the harmful effects of these drugs can be and how much it is safe for a child or an adult to take in one day. You should never take more than the recommended daily dose.

If taken over long periods, some drugs cause people to become psychologically or physically dependent on them. This applies to medicinal drugs as well as to illegal 'street' drugs. Long-term users often suffer very unpleasant side-effects and withdrawal symptoms when they try to stop taking these drugs.

Non-prescription drugs are usually illegal. Alcohol, cigarettes and medicines bought from chemists or supermarkets are the exceptions. People who use 'street' drugs such as heroin, cocaine, marijuana and ecstasy are usually trying to get the short-term feelings of mental pleasure, stimulation and physical energy that the drugs often give. However, in the longer-term all 'street' drugs present major risks to the user's health. They usually have damaging effects on physical health, as well as on social, psychological and financial wellbeing.

OVER TO YOU

How much do you know about the effects and health risks of 'street' drugs? Improve your knowledge and understanding by finding out about them on these websites:

www.teenagehealthfreak.com

www.trashed.co.uk

www.drugworld.org.uk

Print off, or make notes about, the possible health effects of the main 'street' drugs that you investigate.

Solvents are chemical substances made for industrial and scientific use. They are used in the production of cleaning fluids, ink, glue, aerosols and cigarette lighter fuel. People who misuse them are typically teenagers or young adults. Solvent misuse has a number of bad effects on health:

- Cigarette lighter fuel (butane gas) sprayed in the mouth cools the throat tissues causing swelling, and sometimes suffocation.
- Some solvents contain poisonous substances such as lead.
- Solvent misuse causes people to feel reckless, making users less able to deal with danger.
- Solvents are flammable. There is an increased fire risk if the user is smoking.
- Long-term misuse may cause damage to liver, kidneys, lungs, bone marrow and the nervous system.

Quick Questions

1 Name three 'street' drugs that pose a risk to a person's health.
2 Describe the negative effects that misusing prescription medicine can have on a person's health and wellbeing.
3 Explain how solvent misuse can damage a person's physical health.

OVER TO YOU

You can improve your knowledge and understanding of solvent abuse by looking at the following websites:

www.canban.com

www.re-solve.org

Stress

Too much stress is bad for your health. People often talk about 'feeling stressed' and stress has got a bad reputation with health professionals. **Stress** is a response to the demands made on a person. Where the demands outweigh a person's ability to cope or adapt, they feel under pressure, threatened, tense or strained. This is 'stress'.

Stress has both psychological and physical symptoms

- muscle pain
- headaches
- feeling sick
- trembling
- sweating
- dry throat
- disturbed sleep
- changes in appetite
- stomach upset
- fast pulse rate
- feeling faint or dizzy
- irritability
- poor concentration
- feeling panicky

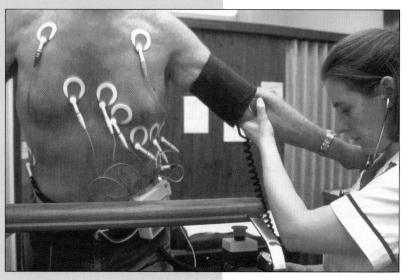

▲ Nurse measuring a patient's blood pressure as he performs exercise during a stress test

Health problems associated with stress

Extreme stress, either sudden or more long-term, produces uncomfortable symptoms and can lead to health problems.

Stress becomes harmful when it is continuous, disrupts everyday life and relationships and becomes too difficult to cope with. Some people experience temporary health problems from which they recover when they manage to reduce their stress levels. For other people, stress has long-term health effects on both their physical and mental health. Stress can trigger mental health problems such as depression and anxiety-based illnesses.

Health problems associated with stress

- anxiety and depression
- eczema
- asthma
- migraine
- angina (pain around the heart muscle)
- high blood pressure
- heart attack
- stomach ulcers
- accidents

Many different factors can cause stress. Exams, assignments, being bullied or being asked questions in class might do it for you. Other common causes of stress in people's lives include relationships, money worries, poor living or work conditions, having too much work to do and general lack of satisfaction in life.

What do you think people can do to reduce or minimise stress? In previous pages, we covered some of the factors that help people to be healthy. Recreation and leisure activity are particularly important for reducing stress levels. Having supportive relationships and satisfying work also helps. Increasingly, people use sports activities to help them to relax and de-stress. Massage, talking to people about problems and feelings, thinking positively and being assertive (saying 'no' to extra work!) are all good ways of reducing stress levels.

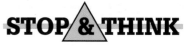

STOP & THINK

Identify three occasions when you've felt very stressed. What were your symptoms? What caused your stress? Make a note of these points or discuss them with a colleague in your class.

Unit 2 Promoting health and wellbeing

CASE STUDY

Neville Williams is 37. He wants to retire as a rich and happy man when he's 50. Neville currently puts all his time and energy into running his own plumbing business. He works between 60 and 80 hours a week, often working throughout the weekend when his friends and family take time off. Neville is feeling under a lot of pressure at the moment. He's told his wife that he's getting headaches that don't seem to go away, feels faint at times when he's working and is having trouble sleeping properly. Despite encouragement, Neville is reluctant to go and see his GP (family doctor) and won't take any time off work. Neville hasn't been on holiday for two years, even though his wife and two children went to Spain last year.

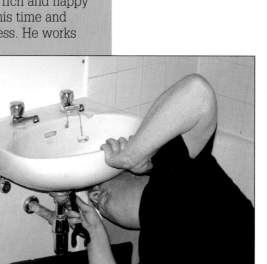

- What symptoms of stress does Neville have?
- What are the possible causes of Neville's current stress problems?
- Explain what might happen to Neville's health and wellbeing if he continues to experience high stress levels?
- Suggest some changes that Neville could be encouraged to make to his life style that would reduce his high stress levels.

Quick Questions

1 Identify three symptoms of stress.
2 Using examples, describe the reasons why teenagers sometimes experience levels of stress that can harm their health or wellbeing.
3 In your own words, explain what 'stress' is.

Personal hygiene

Personal hygiene and body odour (smell) are very sensitive topics for most people. It is not good to be known for your body odour (BO) and bad breath! On the other hand, being clean and smelling pleasant are good for your reputation, social life and self-esteem. In fact, good personal hygiene is an important way of maintaining good health.

A person who fails to maintain good personal hygiene can experience a range of health and social problems. Health problems, such as skin conditions (sores, rashes), result from poor personal hygiene when the bacteria and fungi that naturally grow on, and in, the body are not removed. The body conditions that help bacteria and fungi to grow are:

- moisture from sweat
- warmth from body heat
- food from the dead cells and waste products in sweat.

The areas of the body that need most cleaning are those where sweat is excreted – for example, under the arms, the groin area, the feet, the scalp and hair. Failing to take a daily bath or shower or to wash the skin and clean your teeth, result in a build up of bacteria, dirt and odour.

Acne

Acne (spots, zits, pimples) is something that happens to most teenagers and some adults. Spots are not caused by poor personal hygiene. Cleaning the skin thoroughly and keeping skin pores clear helps to reduce, but cannot prevent, acne. It is caused by hormone imbalances.

Dental hygiene

Health problems can also result from poor dental hygiene. Brushing the teeth properly and using dental floss keeps the teeth clean and helps to prevent decay, gum disease and bad breath.

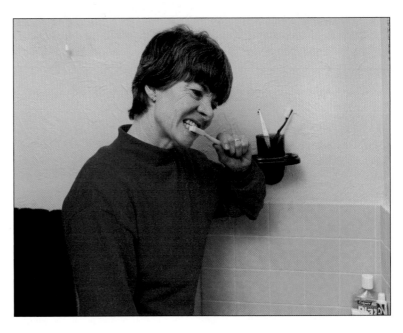

▶ Daily tooth brushing is essential for good dental health

What causes bad breath?

- gum infections
- eating strongly flavoured food like garlic
- rotting teeth
- decaying food stuck between the teeth
- throat infections
- smoking
- not drinking enough water

CASE STUDY

Sandra Davis is the mother of three children. She has just got a job and needs to arrange childcare to cover the time that she and her husband are both at work. You're one of three people who've answered her advert for a childminder for Dion, aged three months, Jay, aged six, and Sonia, aged nine.

In the interview, Sandra explains the arrangements. The children will arrive at your house at about 8.30 a.m. Sandra will pick them up again after work at 4 p.m. Sandra's next questions is: 'What will you do to ensure that each of my children maintains good personal hygiene throughout the day?'

Write an answer explaining what you think the priorities are and indicate what you would do to set and maintain standards of good hygiene practice for each child.

Not looking after your personal hygiene can lead to health problems, such as skin infections. However, the social problems that result from being smelly and unclean are just as great. Personal hygiene problems will have a negative effect on a person's relationships and social life. This is likely to lead to the person feeling rejected, isolated and having low self-esteem.

Quick Questions

1 Identify the main biological causes of body odour.

2 Describe ways in which poor personal hygiene can have a negative effect on a person's social and emotional wellbeing.

3 Explain how a regular personal hygiene routine reduces the risk of ill-health.

Unprotected sex

Everybody has sexual needs. People have sex for a variety of reasons. These include having babies, having orgasms and expressing sexual needs and feelings. Sex isn't terrible, dirty or dangerous. However, choosing to be sexually active does have consequences. These consequences may affect both physical health and emotional wellbeing. The main health risk of sexual activity is from sexually transmitted diseases.

There are at least thirty different types of sexually transmitted disease. Each year they affect about one million men and women in the United Kingdom. Sexually transmitted diseases are caught by having unprotected sex with an infected person. A person can become infected with a sexually transmitted disease after a single act of unprotected sex with another infected person. Young, sexually active people are most at risk of catching a sexually transmitted disease.

The most common sexually transmitted disease is chlamydia. It can cause serious problems such as pelvic inflammatory disease (PID) and inflammation of the oviducts (fallopian tubes) if it is not treated. However, it isn't fatal. People recover after treatment. The table below summarises some of the different types of sexually transmitted diseases and their symptoms.

All diagnoses and workload at genito-urinary medicine clinics, by country: 1995-2000

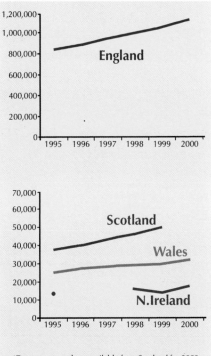

*Data are currently unavailable from Scotland for 2000 and from N.Ireland for 1996 &1997

Girls
- A vaginal discharge that is thick or smelly, has a different colour, is more copious than usual or causes itching may indicate you have thrush*, or trichomoniasis.

- If it hurts when you pass urine (water), you may have cystitis (inflammation of the bladder) or thrush*.

- If your vagina itches or gets sore, you may have thrush*.

- If you develop warty lumps around your vagina or anus (back passage), you may have genital warts.

* Thrush is not always transmitted sexually. The fungus that causes it normally lives in your mouth and vagina. It's kept under control by bacteria in these areas. These natural body defences can be upset by certain illnesses and taking antibiotics or hormones, such as the contraceptive pill. When this happens, you may get thrush.

Boys
- If blood or a discharge comes out of your penis, or passing urine (water) is painful, it may mean you have gonorrhoea, non-specific urethritis or chlamydia.

- If you get warty lumps on or near your penis or anus (back passage), you may have genital warts.

- If you get painful sores or blisters on or near your penis or anus (back passage), you may have herpes.

- If the tip of your penis or area around your anus (back passage)is red and itchy, you may have thrush*.

- If your scrotum and pubic hair are itchy, you may have crabs (pubic lice – small wingless insects that live in pubic hair and feed on blood).

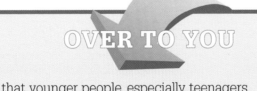

Use medical reference books or a website such as www.teenagehealthfreak.com or www.surgerydoor.co.uk to find out more about the causes, symptoms and consequences of the sexually transmitted diseases referred to above.

OVER TO YOU

HIV and AIDS

The newest and most challenging sexually transmitted disease is the human immunodeficiency virus (**HIV**). This is the virus that causes acquired immune deficiency syndrome (AIDS). If the virus, a simple living organism, gets into the bloodstream it attacks and destroys the body's natural defence mechanisms. An infected person can transmit (pass on) HIV through three different routes:

- sexual intercourse (anal or vaginal)
- blood donation
- drug abuse when non-sterile needles are shared.

By the end of 1998, there had been 11,396 AIDS-related deaths in the United Kingdom and, in total, nearly 50,000 people were reported to have been infected by the HIV virus.

People who do not use condoms and spermicides during sex run a higher risk of catching sexually transmitted diseases and of suffering the various health consequences. Unprotected sex, involving anal or vaginal penetration, allows the release of infected semen or the transfer of vaginal secretions into the body.

OVER TO YOU

Why do you think that younger people, especially teenagers, take risks with sex? Discuss this in a small group and then compare your ideas with those of other groups in the class. Make a list of the most common reasons discussed in the various groups.

Quick Questions

1 Name three sexually transmitted diseases beginning with 'c'.

2 Describe two ways in which a person can minimise the risk of catching a sexually transmitted disease.

3 Explain what the statistics on sexually transmitted diseases reveal about infection patterns within the population of the United Kingdom.

Unemployment and health

Unemployment is something that people of working age worry about and hope they can avoid. A person is unemployed when they don't have work. How do you think it would feel to be unemployed? Losing a job or not being able to obtain work has a variety of effects on people. Few of them are positive. Many older workers dread the prospect of losing their jobs when they reach their forties and fifties. This is because it is so hard for older workers to get work. Older workers often complain that they suffer from age discrimination in the job market.

OVER TO YOU

How would you feel if an employer told you that, despite all your efforts and your good, conscientious service to them, they were very sorry but your services were no longer needed? Write down a few words that you think would describe your emotions. Think about how you would feel about yourself as well as how you would feel about the way that you'd been treated by the employer.

But why is unemployment such a bad thing? Wouldn't you like lots of free time and not to have to get up in the morning to go to work? These things might be good in the short term and you might feel a little like you do when you're on holiday. You could relax with no pressures or timetables to keep to. But this feeling probably wouldn't last long.

People who experience unemployment generally don't feel like they're on holiday. Work is an important source of self-esteem. People take pride in and get status from their jobs. Work plays an important role in our emotional and mental health. Work also provides the money that pays the bills. Not having work has the opposite effect. Unemployed people complain that they feel they don't 'fit in', find themselves outside of their normal social groups and they feel a sense of failure and rejection as a result of not having work. Financial problems occur very quickly when people have no income. All of these consequences can be

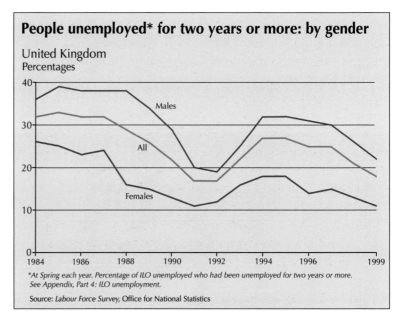

People unemployed* for two years or more: by gender

United Kingdom
Percentages

**At Spring each year. Percentage of ILO unemployed who had been unemployed for two years or more.
See Appendix, Part 4: ILO unemployment.*

Source: *Labour Force Survey*, Office for National Statistics

very damaging if a person experiences long-term unemployment. For example, people can feel hopeless, lose motivation and self-confidence and use harmful substances such as tobacco or alcohol to cope with the negative feelings they experience. Unemployment leads to emotional strain, anxiety and depression and a reduced sense of wellbeing and purpose.

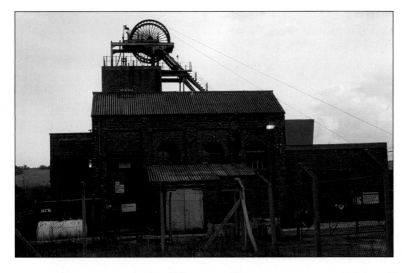

◄ Unemployment rates soared when traditional industries closed down in the 1980s

Unemployment can also have an effect on a person's physical health. Long-term unemployed people are more likely to suffer from respiratory problems, alcohol-related disease, arthritis and mental illness. The connection between these illnesses and unemployment are not clear. Do people become ill because they are unemployed? Or do their illnesses cause them to remain unemployed? Perhaps the lifestyle adopted by unemployed people is less healthy than that of people in work. One of the more common explanations is that unemployment is highly stressful. A high level of personal stress has a negative effect on a person's physical and mental health, their sense of emotional wellbeing and their relationships with others. Without adequate support and strategies to use their time constructively and without the hope of finding work or other fulfilling activity, unemployment will damage a person's health and wellbeing.

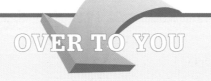

OVER TO YOU

Unemployment usually means a person has a lower income than if they were in work. Explain how this direct effect of unemployment might have an indirect or knock-on effect on an individual's health and wellbeing. Think about the things that people need money for and what might have to be sacrificed if income is reduced.

Quick Questions

1 Identify two aspects of a person's wellbeing that can be affected by unemployment.

2 Describe ways in which unemployment can have an impact on physical health.

3 Analyse possible reasons why the experience of unemployment has little or no impact on some people's health and wellbeing, but a significant effect on others.

Poor housing and health

A person's housing provides them with physical shelter and protection. This is important for physical health. Our accommodation is also emotionally important. The place where you live and spend most of your time is usually more than just somewhere to stay and keep warm and dry. 'Home' provides people with a sense of emotional wellbeing and psychological security. This gives us insight into why poor housing can affect health and wellbeing.

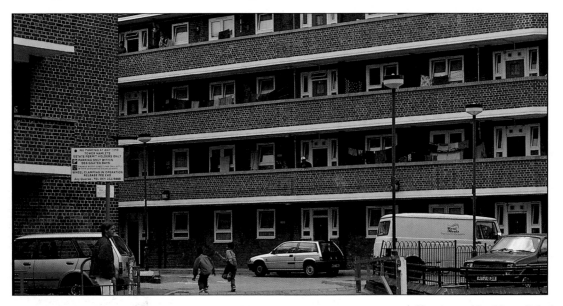

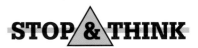
▲ Housing and health are linked.
Where would you prefer to live? ▶

Poor housing can have a direct effect on a person's physical health. For example, lack of adequate heating, dampness and overcrowding can lead to respiratory disorders, stress and mental health problems. Lack of basic amenities, such as a shower or bath; sharing facilities, such as a kitchen or bathroom, between too many people; and cold, damp or unsafe buildings make some people's homes unfit to live in, and may lead to health problems. Lack of security, too much noise and lack of privacy can lead to high stress levels and loss of wellbeing.

Cold and damp housing can aggravate many medical conditions, including asthma, bronchitis and other respiratory diseases, and rheumatism and arthritis. These conditions affect people of all ages, but are particularly unpleasant for babies, infants and older people. Older people with low incomes sometimes have to choose between buying food and heating their homes. The consequence of not having enough heating can be hypothermia (a fall in body temperature to below 35°C – normal body temperature is 37°C).

STOP & THINK

What type of area would you like to live in? Perhaps in a city, or in the country, or by the sea? Identify the type of area you think would make you a happy and healthy person and explain your reasoning.

Overcrowding encourages the spread of infection and infectious diseases such as tuberculosis and dysentery. Children who live in overcrowded homes are more likely to be victims of accidents. Sleeplessness and stress are also associated with overcrowding.

People living in high-rise tower blocks or bedsits may suffer from poor emotional wellbeing because of social isolation. This in turn can lead to low self-esteem and depression. High-rise blocks of flats were built in the United Kingdom during the 1950s and 60s, when there was an acute housing need. The government's long-term plan is now to phase these buildings out and gradually replace them with more appealing housing that is suitable for the wider community. Most housing blocks built in the last few years do not extend beyond four floors.

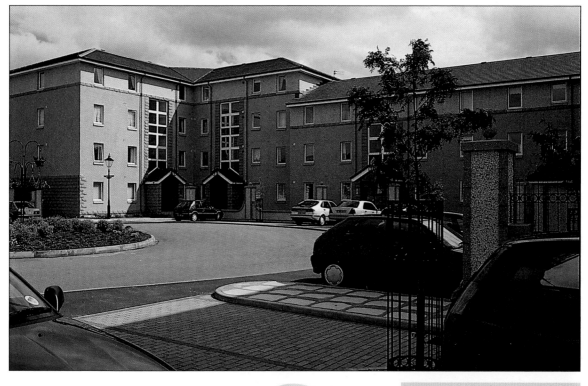

OVER TO YOU

What is healthy housing? Identify the features you feel are important in making a person's housing 'healthy'. Alternatively, identify the negative features that you would look out for if you were house or flat-hunting. Explain, in terms of their effect on health and wellbeing, why you would try to avoid housing that had these negative features.

Quick Questions

1 Which aspect of health and wellbeing is directly affected by inadequate housing?

2 Describe the main features of inadequate housing that are linked to health problems.

3 Explain the link between housing and emotional wellbeing.

Environmental pollution

On page 128 we touched on the idea of living in a 'healthy' area. One of the reasons you may have given when you chose an ideal area to live in might have been clean air, or lack of pollution. Environmental pollution is bad for physical health and most people try to avoid it, if at all possible.

Pollution happens when our natural surroundings (including the air, water and landscape) are contaminated with poisonous or harmful substances. Usually, though not always, this involves the release of high concentrations of a substance, such as chemicals or human sewage. Environmental pollution can remain in the environment for a long time, causing health problems for whole populations for many years.

Pollutants can affect the air, sea, waterways and land. Factories and cars that produce carbon-based fumes are common sources of air pollution. Often we think about only the smoke and fumes that we can see in the environment. However, other air pollutants are less visible. For example, 'acid rain' is ordinary rainwater that has become acidic because it picks up residues of sulphur and nitrogen oxides that are produced by cars, power stations and other factories, often long distances away from where the rain falls. Acid rain is thought to make respiratory problems, such as asthma, worse because it irritates surface membranes in the lungs.

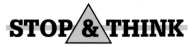

STOP & THINK

Can you think of sources of environmental pollution that affect your everyday surroundings? Identify as many as possible. Think about pollution of the air, water and general environment.

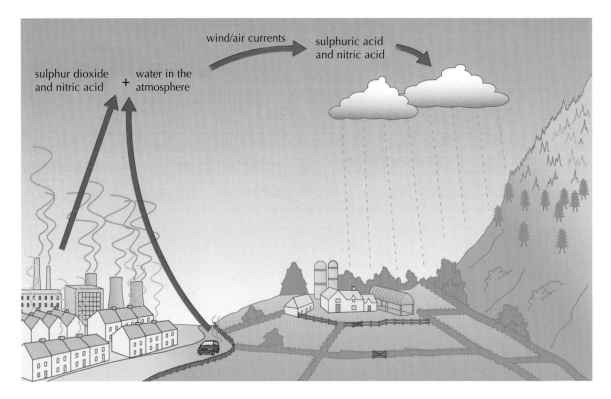

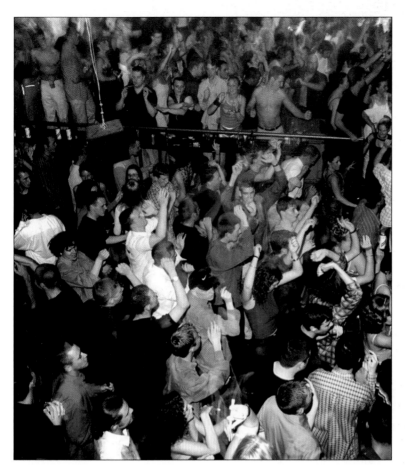

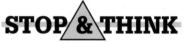

STOP & THINK

Life in the twenty-first century is fast and noisy. What do you think counts as 'noise pollution'? How do you think that excessive or long-term noise pollution could affect a person's health and wellbeing?

You may also have heard about 'greenhouse gases' and the 'ozone layer'. Greenhouse gases are chemicals which, when released into the atmosphere, reduce the thickness of the natural ozone layer. The ozone is a layer of oxygen high in the atmosphere that acts as a thick sunscreen protecting us from the sun's harmful ultraviolet light, which can cause skin cancers. Greenhouse gases can even make holes in this protective layer, increasing our risk of getting skin cancer

Water pollution is usually associated with the release of chemicals, such as oil spills, or untreated human sewage directly into the sea or the domestic water supply. Contaminated water is a particular risk to human health because many infectious diseases are water-borne. These can be quickly spread within a population that is dependent on the infected water source. A contaminated water supply was the cause of numerous outbreaks of infectious epidemics, such as typhoid fever, in the Middle Ages and in the nineteenth century, before sewage treatment became a part of everyday life in the United Kingdom.

Quick Questions

1 Identify two source of air pollution.
2 Describe the possible health effects of water pollution.
3 Explain how forms of pollution can lead to specific health damage.

Build Your Learning

═══ LEARNING POINTS ═══

The following are the main points that you should have learnt from the previous 21 pages.

- A number of factors put an individual's health and wellbeing at risk.

- Risk factors can affect an individual's physical health as well as intellectual, emotional or social wellbeing. Often a risk factor has an impact on more than one area of health and wellbeing.

- Some risks to health and wellbeing result from lifestyle choices that people make. Smoking cigarettes and lack of exercise are examples of health risks that the individual chooses.

- Other risks to health, such as environmental pollution and inherited disease are outside the individual's control. As individuals we may not be able to change the impact of these factors on our health and wellbeing.

REVISION QUESTIONS

If you're confident that you understand the learning points and the key terms, try answering the revision questions below:

1 What are the health risks of:
   a) excess alcohol?
   b) solvent sniffing?
   c) continuous, long-term stress?
   d) unprotected sex?

2 Describe the negative effects on physical health of smoking cigarettes on a regular basis.

3 Explain how a person's lifestyle choices can have a negative effect on their health and wellbeing.

The key question that you should be able to answer if you've understood the previous section is:

4 'What factors are risks to health and wellbeing and how do they have a damaging effect?' Write an answer in your own words.

KEY TERMS

You should know what the following terms mean:

- Inherited disease (page 112)
- Genes (page 112)
- Nicotine (page 114)
- Tar (page 114)
- Haemoglobin (page 114)
- Carbon monoxide (page 114)
- Coronary heart disease (page 115)
- Cirrhosis (page 117)
- Drug misuse (page 118)
- Solvents (page 119)
- Stress (page 120)
- Sexually transmitted disease (page 124)
- Chlamydia (page 124)
- Cystitis (page 124)
- Genital warts (page 124)
- Gonorrhoea (page 124)
- Crabs (page 124)
- Herpes (page 124)
- Thrush (page 124)
- HIV (page 125)
- Unemployment (page 126)
- Pollution (page 130)

If you're not sure or want to check your understanding, turn to the page number listed in the brackets.

INVESTIGATION IDEAS

1 Investigate a genetically inherited condition. You can get information from sources such as library books, the internet and voluntary organisations working with people who have the condition. Produce a summary of causes of the condition and its effects on a person's health and development throughout their life.

2 Try to find out how much housing and environmental conditions have changed in your local area over the last 50 years. You might find this information in history books, the local history section in the public library or by talking to older people who've lived in the area since they were children.

3 Search the archives of online newspapers, such as the Electronic Telegraph (www.telegraph.co.uk) and the Guardian (www.guardian.co.uk), to find information on the causes and health effects of environmental disasters, such as the Chernobyl nuclear accident in the USSR or the Bhopal chemical accident in India.

We've already looked at various factors affecting a person's health and wellbeing. These included factors such as exercise and a balanced diet, that promote good health, and cigarette smoking which doesn't. But how can we know whether a person is healthy or not? One way is to measure specific aspects (indicators) of their physical health. In this section, you will learn how these indicators can be measured and how they are used to assess the state of an individual's physical health. The measures we'll consider are:

- blood pressure
- peak flow (breathing out)
- body mass index
- pulse (at rest, and on recovery after exercise).

▲ Which aspect of health is being measured here?

The information in this section will help you to understand how and why physical health is measured. It won't teach you how to make these measures. The techniques used to measure physical health are skills that health professionals learn both during their training and on the job.

How can physical health be measured?

You've probably had aspects of your physical health measured many times. This will have happened when you visited your GP (family doctor) or if you've ever been to hospital for assessment or treatment. You've probably also watched television programmes set in hospitals where the staff seem to spend a lot of time checking the state of their patients' health and worrying over the dramatic results.

So, how do health care workers tell if a person is physically healthy or not? There are, in fact, many different ways of measuring physical health. They are all based on the same basic idea – the health care worker measures and records something and then compares the individual's 'score' against a standard scale. But what do they measure?

Measuring the pulse rate

The pulse rate, both before and after exercise, is often used to determine a person's general health or physical fitness. The **pulse rate** indicates how fast the heart is beating. For adults, the average (or normal) resting rate is usually between 70 and 80 beats per minute. Babies and young children normally have a faster pulse rate than adults.

The pulse can be felt at any artery. In conscious people, it is usual to use the **radial artery**, which can be felt at the wrist. In unconscious people, the **carotid artery**, which can be felt at the neck, may be used. (Most conscious people would find it uncomfortable if you pressed on their carotid artery!) Pulse rate increases when you exercise, when you're emotionally upset or if you develop a form of heart or respiratory disease. People who are unfit, who smoke cigarettes or who are overweight have a faster resting pulse rate than normal.

▲ Measuring the radial pulse

▶ Measuring the carotid pulse

Measure your own, or another person's, pulse rate (using the radial pulse!) for one minute. Compare the resting pulse rate with the pulse rate taken after some brief exercise.

OVER TO YOU

Measuring blood pressure

Health professionals routinely measure their patient's blood pressure as well as their pulse rate. Blood pressure measurement is a direct way of checking heart functioning, and indirectly physical fitness.

But what does blood pressure measure? **Blood pressure** is a measure of two things. First, it is the force, or pressure, which the blood puts on the walls of the artery when the heart beats. Second, it is the pressure that blood continuously puts on the arteries between heart beats.

Blood pressure should only be measured by a qualified and experienced health care professional. It is measured with an instrument called a **sphygmomanometer** or 'sphyg' for short. Some health professionals use electronic sphygs which measure automatically and display the results on a screen. The other way of measuring blood pressure is to use a manual sphyg.

A manual sphyg consists of an inflatable cuff connected via a rubber tube to a column of mercury with a graduated scale. The cuff is placed around the person's arm and gently inflated until it stops blood flow through the brachial artery. (The radial pulse in the same arm will also temporarily disappear.) As the pressure cuff is inflated the column of mercury rises on the display.

At the same time, the health professional uses a stethoscope, with the diaphragm placed over the brachial artery where it passes inside the elbow, to listen to the changing sounds made as the pulse beat disappears from, and later returns to, the artery.

The pressure cuff is then slowly deflated until the health professional hears the first sound of blood re-entering the artery. The health professional notes the value on the column of mercury at which this happened. This sound is caused each time the heart pumps blood out around the body and is known as the **systolic blood pressure**.

The cuff is then gradually deflated until all sounds disappear. The point at which the last beat is heard
is known as the **diastolic blood pressure**. This measures the continuous pressure of the blood in the arteries.

Blood pressure is measured in millimetres of mercury. On average it measures 120/80 mm Hg (millimetres of mercury) in the young adult.

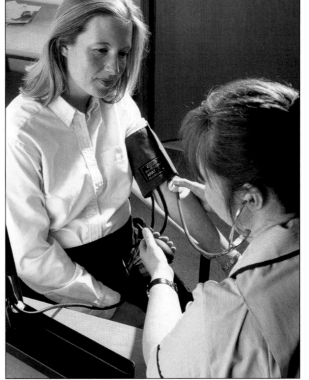

▲ Measuring blood pressure using a manual sphygmomanometer

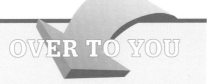

OVER TO YOU

Find out what effect each of the following has on a person's blood pressure:

- a diet high in fat and salt
- regular exercise
- stress
- cigarette smoking

Find out the difference between hypertension and hypotension.

Quick Questions

1 Identify the main methods of measuring a person's heart rate.

2 Using your own words, explain what the systolic and diastolic numbers in a blood pressure figure are measuring.

3 Explain what a high diastolic measurement would tell you about a person's blood pressure.

Measuring respiratory health

A person's respiratory health (breathing) can be assessed by recording simple physical measurements. Respiratory health can be measured by using a peak flow meter. You may have seen or used a peak flow meter, especially if you have asthma or have had other respiratory health checks.

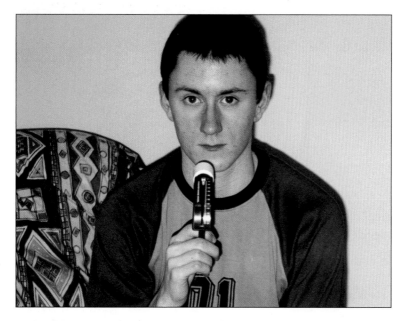

◀ Peak flow meters are easy to use

A peak flow meter measures the maximum rate at which air is expelled (pushed out) from the lungs when a person breathes out as hard as they can. The peak flow meter is one example of a pulmonary (lung) function test. These tests are used to monitor several aspects of respiratory function. For example, the peak flow meter can be used to diagnose whether a person has a problem with the use of their lungs, because there is a standard scale of expected scores against which the results can be compared. People with chronic (long-term) asthma usually record a measurement that is lower than 350 on the peak-flow scale.

Measuring body mass

In adults, the relationship between height and weight can be an indicator of good or ill health. Health professionals recommend that a person's weight should be in proportion to his or her height (see the height and weight chart on the opposite page). A person is considered obese when his or her weight is more than 20 per cent above the average weight for people of the same height and similar personal and cultural characteristics. People whose weight is much greater than that recommended for them run the risk of developing a range of health problems.

Health problems associated with obesity
- arthritis
- high blood pressure
- increased risk of stroke
- diabetes
- gallstones
- heart disease

Health professionals use the **body mass index** (BMI) to assess whether a person is underweight, normal, overweight or obese. This involves more than just measuring weight. You can use the following formula to work out your BMI.

Body mass index is calculated by dividing your weight in kilograms by your height in metres squared. This will give you a number which you should compare to the following categories:

BMI	Category
Below 20	Underweight
20-25	Normal
25-30	Overweight
Over 30	Obese

Height and weight charts are also used by health professionals, and people interested in their own health, to measure and assess whether their weight is within the normal, healthy range. You might like to try using this height/ weight chart.

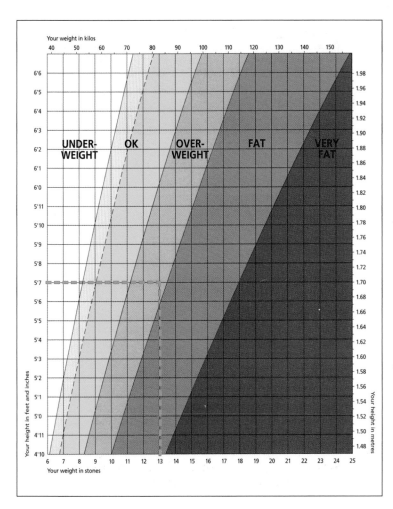

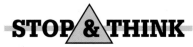

STOP & THINK

Is your BMI within or outside of the normal range? If outside, how can you adjust your health-related behaviour to bring it within the normal, healthy range?

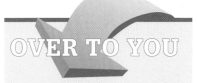

OVER TO YOU

You can find more information on weight, BMI and weight measurement on several websites. Try those listed below or carry out a search of your own:

www.teenagehealthfreak.com

www.surgerydoor.co.uk

www.weightlossresources.co.uk

Some of the sites will calculate your BMI for you if you know your height and weight measurements.

Quick Questions

1 Identify the two measures needed to calculate a person's body mass index (BMI).

2 Describe the possible impact of obesity on an individual's health and wellbeing.

3 Explain the purpose and use of a peak flow meter.

CASE STUDY

Chris Henry was very fit during his early twenties. He remembers going to the gym a couple of times a week, playing football at weekends and, at 30, he even ran thirteen miles in a half-marathon. Chris is now 45. He's become overweight and unfit during the last ten years. He says this has happened because he's stopped taking part in sport and also he drinks and smokes more than he used to. Chris is now very keen to improve his health generally and his physical fitness in particular. He realises that he'll never be as fit as he was in his twenties, but thinks that losing two stone in weight and improving his stamina will benefit his health.

1 Identify the baseline measures that should be taken before Chris begins his health improvement plan.

2 Suggest three health targets that could be a part of Chris's health improvement plan.

3 What types of exercise would you recommend for Chris as a way of reducing his weight and improving his stamina?

4 Apart from increasing the amount of exercise he does, how else could Chris change his lifestyle to reach his health improvement goals?

Build Your Learning

LEARNING POINTS

The following are the main points that you should have learnt from the previous six pages.

- Some indicators of a person's physical health can be measured. These include pulse, peak flow, blood pressure and body mass index .

- Pulse and body mass can be measured without the need for equipment or special training. Blood pressure and peak flow should only be measured by trained care workers with access to appropriate equipment.

- Health professionals assess how physically healthy a person is by comparing their individual measurements against standard or 'average' measurements for similar people within the population.

- Several factors, which include, age, sex and lifestyle, have to be taken into account when assessing whether a person's pulse, peak flow, body mass index or blood pressure are within the 'normal' range.

KEY TERMS

You should know what the following terms mean:

- Blood pressure (page 134)
- Pulse rate (page 134)
- Radial artery (page 134)
- Carotid artery (page 134)
- Sphygmomanometer (page 134)
- Systolic blood pressure (page 135)
- Diastolic blood pressure (page 135)
- Peak flow meter (page 136)
- Body mass index (page 137)

If you're not sure or want to check your understanding, turn to the page number listed in the brackets.

REVISION QUESTIONS

If you're confident that you understand the learning points and the key terms, try answering the revision questions below:

1 What's the difference between:
   a) peak flow and pulse?

   b) blood pressure and body mass index?

   c) systolic and diastolic blood pressure?

   d) being overweight and being obese?

2 Describe how a person's blood pressure is measured manually by a health professional.

3 Explain why a high body mass index (BMI) should be a cause for concern.

The key question that you should be able to answer if you've understood the previous section is:

4 'How can an individual's physical health be measured?' Have a go at answering this, using your own words.

Have you ever set yourself a goal of 'being healthier' or 'getting fit'. A common time to do this is just after Christmas, when people often feel they've had too much to eat or drink. We've probably all wanted to improve our health and wellbeing at one time or another. However, health improvement needs to be based on more than good intentions, joining a gym or walking a bit more than we usually do. In the following pages we look at ways of planning health improvement and how we can set realistic and achievable health targets.

The area of care practice that focuses on health improvement is known as health promotion work, or health education work. Health promotion involves providing information containing 'health messages' to individuals, to various social groups, to a whole community or, on a larger scale, to the general public. The aim of health promotion activity is to provide people with information and advice on ways of raising their health status and sense of wellbeing.

Health promotion campaigns

▼ A doctor's surgery notice board showing examples of some health promotion activities

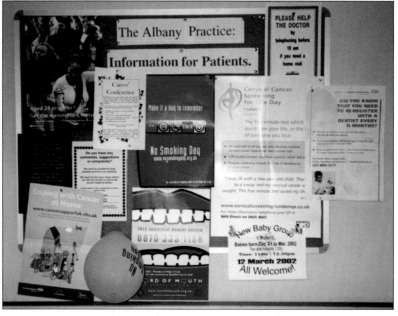

Many large-scale health promotion campaigns, such as the Christmas anti-drink–driving campaigns, are carried out by government agencies. You've probably seen examples of various campaigns in newspapers and magazines, on television or in booklets and posters. You may have come across them at your local leisure centre, sports ground, health centre, library, shopping centre, health food shop, school, college, hospital, nursery or youth club.

Large-scale health promotion work is an important way of getting health messages to large groups of people. This may mean to everyone in the United Kingdom. However, large-scale health promotion isn't the only type of health promotion work. Health promotion is also targeted on a smaller scale at individuals and small groups. This type of health promotion work is usually done by individual health

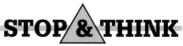

STOP & THINK

Can you think of any health promotion campaigns that you've seen? Where did you see the information? How did it affect you?

professionals, for example doctors and nurses, during their work with patients. A care worker may have given you, or somebody you know, advice or guidance on ways of improving your health or sense of wellbeing. 'Do more exercise' and 'stop smoking' often form part of a health promotion 'message'.

Health promotion work involves more than just giving bits of advice to people. In the next few pages, we look at what is involved in large-scale health promotion work.

STOP & THINK

Can you think of the last time that a health professional gave you advice or information that was designed to improve your physical health or wellbeing?

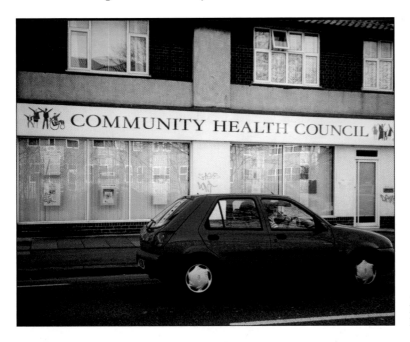

◀ Community Health Councils provide local people with information about health services

Providing health information

Careful planning and preparation are essential for successful large-scale health promotion work. This type of work is usually carried out by a team of people employed as **health promotion officers**. When the team needs to give health promotion messages (a campaign) to the public about topics such as drug misuse, smoking or exercise, it must:

- clearly identify the target group
- identify the key aims (what it wants to do) and objectives (what it wants to achieve) of the campaign
- decide on the best way of putting the key messages across
- identify the resources needed to deliver the messages
- decide how the effectiveness of the campaign will be evaluated (this is feedback – finding out if the public received, understood and acted on the message).

Quick Questions

1 Give an example of a health promotion campaign that is run regularly using TV and radio adverts.

2 Describe the main purpose of large-scale health promotion activity.

3 Explain how a team of health promotion officers would approach the planning and preparation of a large-scale health promotion campaign.

Targeting advice and information

Health promotion campaigns are usually designed to reach specific groups in the population, known as **target groups**. The following social groups are often the target of health promotion activity:

- teenagers
- young people
- pregnant women
- smokers
- people who are obese
- people who have an alcohol problem
- homeless people
- travellers
- pre-retirement groups.

OVER TO YOU

Why do you think that these groups are often targeted with health promotion messages? Think about one or two of them and try to work out reasons why they might be chosen. Write your ideas down. Do the groups have anything in common that might explain why they are the target of health promotion activity?

When planning a health promotion campaign for a specific group, the reasons for the campaign must be clearly identified from the outset. Reasons could be:

- to provide advice and support
- to supply information
- to help people to change or modify their health-related behaviour.

CASE STUDY

Vicky is a district nurse. She visits a large number of older people who live alone in their own homes and are cared for by relatives or partners. When Vicky visits, these carers often complain to her about a range of health problems of their own, such as back pain, depression and stress. Vicky is considering how to begin some health promotion work with this group of socially isolated carers.

- Who is the target group for Vicky's health promotion work?
- What reason's can you think of for carrying out health promotion work with this group?

What topics do health promotion workers provide advice and information about? Sometimes they choose areas of behaviour or factors that are a risk to health. These include smoking, obesity, exercise, alcohol and drug misuse. Unprotected sex, especially its links to HIV infection, has been the subject of many large-scale health promotion campaigns.

Health promotion activity isn't just about health dangers and giving warnings. Increasingly it is about promoting positive health.
You may see health promotion activities that focus on:

- how to lose weight safely and quickly
- how to get the most from local health services
- how to lead an active life after disability
- ways of keeping warm in winter
- healthy eating
- preparation for retirement
- the benefits of exercise
- maintaining personal hygiene
- preventing dental problems
- getting the best out of sport and leisure facilities
- how to maintain desired weight in pregnancy.

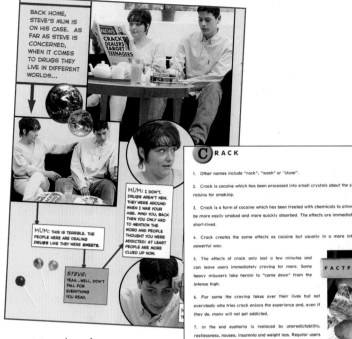

▲ The same health promotion message may be delivered quite differently to different target groups

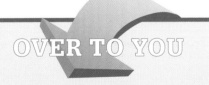
OVER TO YOU

Teenagers are very sensitive about being 'told what to do' even if this is intended as health promotion advice. Imagine that you are a health promotion officer. You've been asked to:

- Identify three key health topics affecting teenagers.
- Suggest a health message for each topic about which teenagers ought to be aware.
- Propose a way of getting each health message across to the teenage target group.

Think about this health promotion challenge and write down your suggestions.

Quick Questions

1 Identify three health promotion target groups.

2 Suggest one health-related topic about which each of your three target groups should be informed.

3 Explain why health promotion workers need to be both persuasive and sensitive in the way they approach health topics.

Choosing campaign methods

Health promotion campaigns are more effective if they are well prepared. The best method of getting the key messages of the campaign across needs to be identified. Health promotion workers make use of a variety of methods including:

- poster campaigns
- television and radio campaigns
- talks and lectures
- seminars
- workshops
- information films and videos
- information packs
- booklets and leaflets
- games and role plays
- promotional displays.

The health promotion team must choose the delivery method that will be most effective in reaching its particular target group, and also in getting the key health message across.

Aged 24 or under? Get the meningitis C message

ⓘmmunisation
the safest way to protect your health

OVER TO YOU

Adverts and promotional campaigns aim to deliver a distinctive message. Some do this in subtle ways, others do it in very strong, obvious ways. They try to persuade the person reading or watching the message either to do something or to think about something.

1 Make a list of the features you believe are important in making communications such as adverts and health campaigns persuasive.

2 What is your favourite advertisement or health campaign? Identify it and describe the features you like and which you think make it memorable.

CASE STUDY

Men don't often talk to each other about their personal health and wellbeing. They are also less likely than women to visit their GP (family doctor), if they do have health concerns. This means that some men don't get the appropriate treatment that could limit or cure their problems. Avoiding contact with health care services, and being unaware of disease symptoms, may result in some men developing high-risk conditions, such as testicular cancer, that become untreatable.

- Suggest some aims for a health promotion campaign targeted at men.

- What methods could be used to promote both health awareness and a preventive approach to health with men as the target group? Explain why you would use the methods you choose.

- What barriers would your health promotion campaign have to overcome before it made a difference to men's health?

OVER TO YOU

Choose any one of the following topics to develop a health message targeted at children:

- dental health
- balanced diet
- smoking
- exercise
- personal safety.

1 Identify a message suitable for promoting good health and wellbeing to a group of children aged seven to nine years.

2 Identify the health promotion methods that could be used to get this message across to these children. Explain why you think your methods would be effective.

Quick Questions

1 Identify three ways of delivering health promotion information to children and adults who can't read.

2 Describe an example of health promotion information that you believe is attractive and effective in getting the health message across to the target group.

3 Explain the advantages and disadvantages of using shocking television adverts to deter teenagers from using 'street' drugs such as heroin.

Health improvement planning

Have you ever been on a diet in order to lose weight? Perhaps you've tried to give up smoking, joined a gym or taken up a sport to 'get fit'. All these things are examples of health improvement activities. Newspapers, magazines and television regularly run stories and programmes on ways of improving personal health and fitness. Some people feel very guilty about 'being unhealthy' and, despite trying various ways of improving their health, feel as though they never quite succeed. This is particularly the case with regular dieters. Despite this, the good news is that it is possible to improve your health and wellbeing. The solution is to choose an effective way of doing so rather than to follow the latest diet or fitness fad.

Target setting

Individual health improvement should begin with thorough and honest health assessment. This involves collecting basic health-related information and also measuring physical health indicators.

Information needed for a personal health assessment

- Lifestyle information
- Dietary intake
- Amount of sleep
- Units of alcohol consumed
- Exercise pattern
- Use of cigarettes or drugs
- Physical measures
- Height
- Weight
- Pulse
- Blood pressure

The information collected provides a baseline measure, or starting point, from which to work. One useful way of collecting lifestyle information is to write a health diary for a couple of weeks. This will involve keeping an honest record of what you eat and drink, the amount of sleep you get, your exercise patterns, how many cigarettes you smoke (if any) and any other substances, like alcohol or drugs, that you consume (if any). This diary record, combined with physical measures, enables you to identify some of the factors that may be contributing to a health problem (such as lack of exercise or unbalanced diet) and also provides a basis on which to set realistic improvement targets.

Before you begin setting your health improvement targets, it's important to compare your own physical health measures with those recommended or expected for someone of your age and physical characteristics. Identify the measures (pulse rate, for example) that are outside the expected range, those that match the recommendations and those that are within reasonable limits. You'll then know which areas you need to concentrate on to improve your physical health and wellbeing.

The next stage is to set targets for improvement. You should ensure that your targets are safe, realistic and achievable. Health improvement should be a gradual process. You shouldn't go on 'crash diets' or exercise binges to lose weight rapidly. You'll only gain the weight again and may damage your physical health in the process. You should have a clear and logical plan for setting particular targets. It's best to set short-, medium- and long-term targets, and to build in regular reassessment opportunities, so that you can see how you're getting on.

The methods you use to work towards, and achieve, your health improvement targets should be safe and, ideally, fit in with your current lifestyle. For example, improving physical fitness can be achieved in many different ways. Walking more, cycling to school or going to an exercise class once a week are all relatively straightforward and won't disrupt your lifestyle too much. Setting yourself targets of running a marathon or swimming the English Channel are probably unrealistic and unsafe!

If you need to develop a health improvement plan for another person, remember to take their age and physical characteristics into account when conducting their health assessment. For your plan to succeed in improving their health, they must be motivated and agree both to your plan and to the targets that you've set for them.

Quick Questions

1 Identify three factors that must be assessed before a health improvement plan can be written.

2 Describe how health behaviour and lifestyle can be assessed as part of a health improvement programme.

3 Explain why health assessment is a necessary part of planning health improvement.

OVER TO YOU

Develop a simple but realistic plan for improving your health and wellbeing.

1 Collect information about the health-related aspects of your lifestyle and record your basic physical measures of health. You may want to produce a diary for the first part of this task and get some help in doing the second part.

2 Compare your personal results to those recommended for someone of your age and physical characteristics.

3 Identify those aspects of your health you need to improve and set yourself a couple of short-, medium- and long-term targets.

4 Identify ways of working towards and reaching your targets.

CASE STUDY

Stephen Ganda, is the manager of a leisure centre. Recently, he's noticed that groups of teenagers have started to meet outside the centre. The teenagers seem to spend their time smoking and drinking wine and cans of beer. Stephen has spoken to the teenagers about the situation as he is concerned about the effects of regular drinking and smoking on the teenagers' health and wellbeing. The teenagers say that they're just enjoying themselves and aren't harming anyone. Stephen has decided to approach the local health promotion unit to request that they plan and carry out some health promotion work with the teenagers.

1 Identify the health risks that result from the teenagers behaviour.

2 Which health topic do you think the local health promotion unit should concentrate on?

3 Identify a clear health message that you would want to communicate to the teenagers in a health education campaign.

4 Explain how you would go about getting this health message across to this target group.

CASE STUDY

Angela Perry is a health promotion officer. She has been asked by a local housing estate residents' committee to begin some health promotion work with local young people. They say that the current health issues affecting young people on the estate are teenage pregnancy, alcohol and drug misuse.

1 Choose one of health issues identified by the residents' committee and identify the aims of a health promotion campaign. (Hint – what would you be trying to achieve?)

2 Suggest three different methods that could be used to provide information about your chosen health issue.

3 Describe any problems that you think a health promotion campaign targeted at young people on the estate might face.

4 Suggest ways of overcoming these problems.

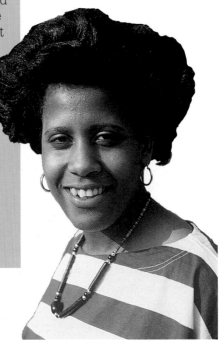

Build Your Learning

KEY TERMS

You should know what the following terms mean:

- Health promotion (page 140)
- Health messages (page 140)
- Health promotion officers (page 141)
- Target groups (page 142)
- Health improvement planning (page 146)
- Target setting (page 146)
- Baseline measure (page 146)

If you're not sure or want to check your understanding, turn to the page number listed in the brackets.

REVISION QUESTIONS

If you're confident that you understand the learning points and the key terms, try answering the revision questions below:

1 What's the difference between:

a) a target group and target-setting?

b) a health promotion campaign and a health improvement plan?

c) a health promotion method and a health promotion message?

2 Describe ways in which health promotion information can be effectively targeted at the general population.

3 Explain why individual health assessment and target setting are essential before an effective health improvement plan can be constructed.

The key question that you should be able to answer if you've understood the previous section is:

4 'How can individuals be motivated and supported to improve their health?' Have a go at answering this.

INVESTIGATION IDEAS

1 Find the location of your local health promotion unit. Arrange to visit, perhaps with some of your class colleagues, or ask a representative to visit your school or college. Find out what local health promotion officers are doing and what campaigns or projects they are currently working on.

2 Visit places in your local area where you would expect to find health promotion information. These might include your GP surgery, local library, a sports centre or a youth club. Try to find examples of health promotion material on display. Have a good look at them and collect any take-away information available. Write a brief report describing the information and explaining who it is aimed at, what the health messages are and whether you think it is effective.

3 Talk to somebody who helps others to 'get fit', such as a PE teacher, a fitness trainer or a fitness-class teacher. Find out from them how they assess fitness, how they set targets and the methods that they use to motivate people to improve their fitness.

Understanding personal development and relationships

This unit is about personal development and relationships across the life span. You will learn about:

- the stages and patterns of human growth and development
- the different factors that can affect human growth and development
- the development of self-concept and personal relationships
- major life changes and how people deal with them
- the role of relationships in personal development.

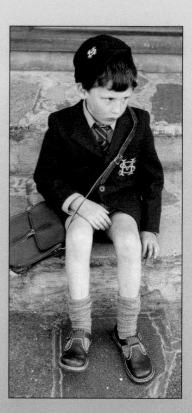

Health and social care workers are employed to work with people of all ages and backgrounds. A clear understanding of how people normally grow and develop during each stage of life is part of the knowledge that care workers need to help people who experience health- and care-related problems. This unit will give you a better understanding of human growth and development and the factors that affect them.

Unit 3 of this book covers Unit 3, Understanding personal development and relationships, of the GCSE Health and Social Care award.

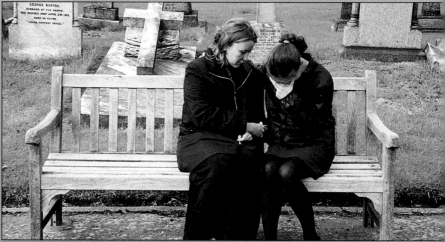

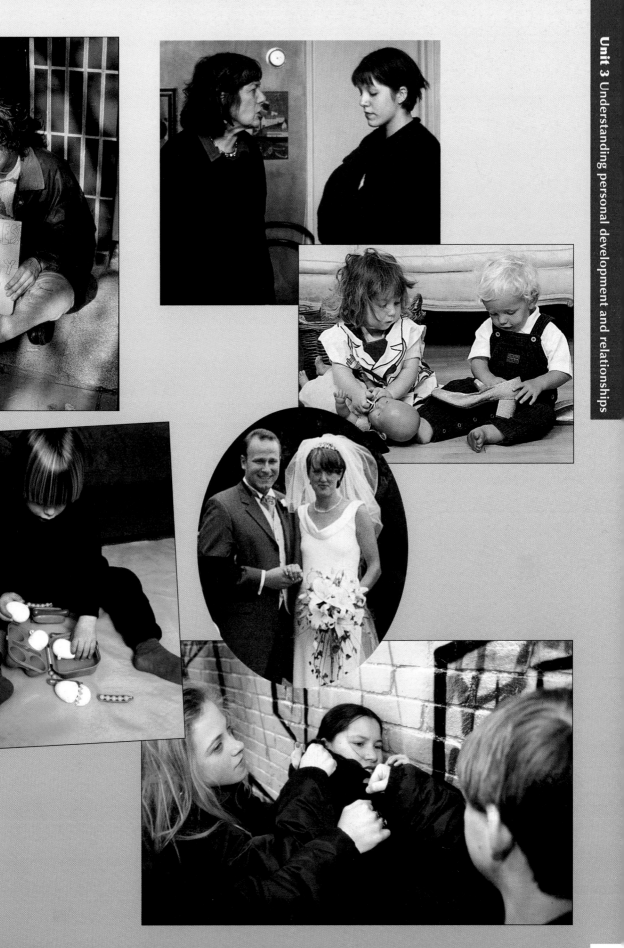

What does human growth and development involve? How is it triggered? Do all people develop in the same way? To understand human growth and development you need to know the meaning of some key ideas that are commonly used by care workers.

Life stages and the life span

People are said to go through a number of life stages during their life span. A **life stage** is a defined period of growth and development. The five main human life stages in which physical growth and personal development occur are:

- infancy (birth–3 years)
- childhood (4–10 years)
- adolescence (11–18 years)
- adulthood (19–65 years)
- later adulthood (65 + years).

These stages cover the whole of the human life span. The **life span** is the time between a person's birth and his or her death. As we saw in unit 2 (see page 106), while all people are living to an increasingly old age, women have a longer life span than men do.

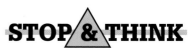

STOP & THINK

What reasons would you give to explain why women tend to live longer than men do?

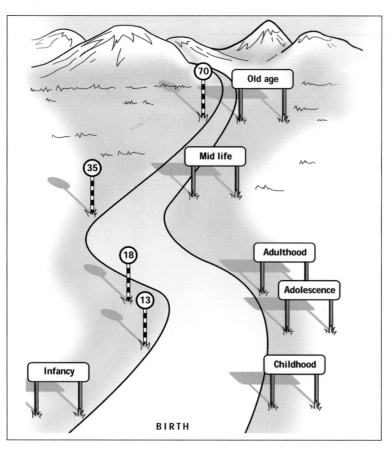

What are 'growth' and 'development'?

The terms 'growth' and 'development' mean different things. **Growth** refers to the increase in physical size, or mass, that occurs as a person gradually moves from infancy through childhood into adulthood. **Development** refers to the way a person acquires new skills and capabilities. A person's skills and abilities become more sophisticated and complex as they progress towards adulthood. People experience most growth and development during infancy, childhood and adolescence.

Within each of the five main life stages, changes occur in our physical, emotional, social, and intellectual characteristics, qualities, and abilities. We will look at examples of these changes later in this unit.

Developmental norms

The ways in which people grow and develop tend to follow a pattern. The growth and development 'milestones' (learning to sit up, walk and talk, for example), and the points in a person's life when they happen are commonly referred to as **developmental norms**.

Examples of developmental norms	
Baby can sit unaided	6 – 9 months
Baby can crawl	8 – 10 months
Baby can walk unaided	12 – 13 months
Infant can say a few words	9 – 12 months
Puberty begins	10 (girl) 12 (boys)
Menopause occurs	45 – 55 years

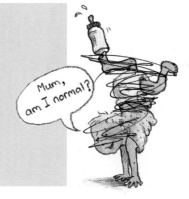

There is a generally expected pattern of human growth and development. Infants, children and adolescents tend to develop particular skills (such as walking) at about the same age. However, it is important not to think of this pattern as an exact timetable that 'normal' people follow. A child, teenager or adult is not abnormal if he or she reaches growth and developmental milestones at slightly different times to the expected pattern. His or her development, whether it is faster or slower than the norm, may be different for a variety of reasons. The general pattern of human development is described in the life stage case studies that appear throughout this unit.

Quick Questions

1 Using your own words, explain what the terms 'growth' and 'development' mean.

2 What does the term 'life span' mean?

3 Name the type of ability that is affected by intellectual development.

Most of the physical growth and change that people experience is predictable and is part of a natural human process of ageing. The **ageing process** refers to the ways in which the human body gradually changes over time.

Physical growth

Human growth is a continuous process. However, the increases that we experience in our physical size (height and weight) tend to occur mainly during infancy, childhood and adolescence. Infancy is a life stage in which a person grows very rapidly. Another growth spurt occurs in adolescence, when we grow to our maximum height. Growth during childhood is usually steady and continuous – making it less noticeable than the growth spurts of infancy or adolescence. While many people do experience physical changes during adulthood (especially in their weight!), most of our natural body-building processes are completed in early adulthood.

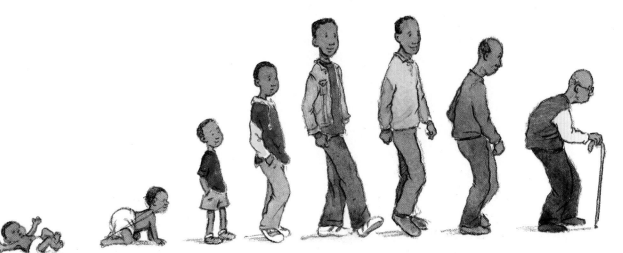

Physical development

Human beings develop physical skills from birth. We experience a peak in our physical ability during adulthood. We then experience a slow, gradual decline in our physical abilities until the point in old age at which we die.

STOP & THINK

Can you think of a physical ability that is first developed during childhood?

The physical changes that occur as we grow older are mainly influenced by **maturation.** This is a lifelong process in which growth and developmental changes occur in sequence. Maturation is thought to be controlled by a biological 'programme' built into our genes, which controls the ageing process. The rate, or speed, at which people age varies. For example, some very old people retain their energy, mental alertness and enjoyment of life longer than other much younger people do. The rate at which people age is influenced by factors such as whether a person inherits 'long life' genes from their parents, their attitude to life, their health and fitness, and the extent to which they live a stressful life.

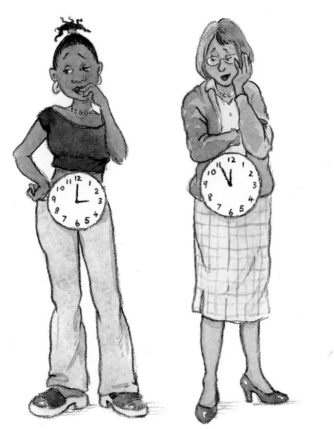

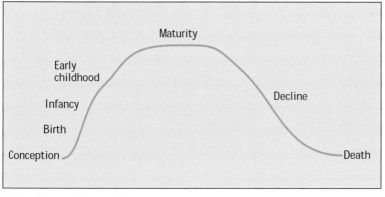

▲ Development is a continuous process

Quick Questions

1 What term is used to describe the process of change that people experience throughout their lives?

2 In which life stage do people experience their last 'growth spurt' and reach their maximum height?

3 Explain, using your own words, what the term 'maturation' means.

The emotional and social aspects of personal development begin at birth and are very closely related to each other. These areas of personal development are concerned with people's feelings (emotional) and relationships (social).

Emotional development

Emotions are feelings, such as love, happiness, disappointment and anger. We develop and express these through our experience of relationships and social situations. People experience emotional development in each life stage. The way that others treat an individual has an effect on their emotional development, whatever life stage they're in. Emotional development involves:

- growth of feelings about and awareness of your 'self'
- growth of feelings towards other people
- development of self-image and identity.

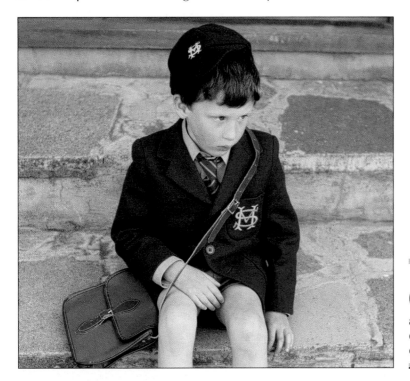

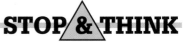

STOP & THINK

Can you remember how you felt on your first day at school? What kinds of emotions did you experience?

Social development

Social development involves the growth of our relationships with others, the social skills we develop and use in relating to others, and learning the culture (or way of life) of the society in which we live. Parents and teachers play a very important part in our social development. They teach us about the acceptable ways of behaving. This involves how we relate to others in everyday situations and the importance of making, and keeping, good relationships with other

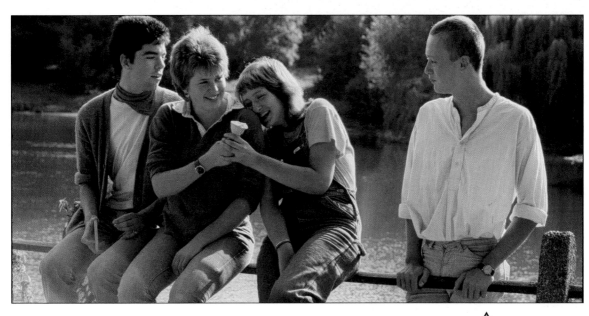

people. Friends and work colleagues are another very important sources of socialisation later in life. Friends are particularly important during later adolescence when we are trying to find and express our own individual identities and forming closer friendships with others.

STOP & THINK

In what ways do your friends help or support you emotionally?

Intellectual development

The term **intellectual development** is used to describe the ways in which thinking, memory and language abilities improve and are refined throughout life. Intellectual development is a process that occurs in all human life stages.

A few centuries ago the belief was that children were born with a mind that was like an empty book. People thought that the 'book' gradually filled up with knowledge and information as the child gained experience in the environment. This view is no longer as popular or widely held as it once was. There are now a number of different ways of explaining intellectual development.

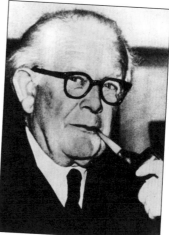

◀ Jean Piaget, a developmental psychologist

Jean Piaget (1896–1980), a Swiss scientist interested in children's development, produced a theory that claims children are born with some basic abilities and lots of intellectual potential. He believed that a person's intellectual potential gradually unfolds as they grow older.

Our intellectual abilities are now thought to be maturing during infancy and childhood. With the help of planned learning experiences in educational settings – such as school, college and university – and also through informal learning in work and social situations, our intellectual abilities are nurtured so that we fulfil our potential.

Quick Questions

1 In which life stage does language development improve rapidly?

2 What factors are said to influence a person's emotional development?

3 Identify the groups of people who play an important role in social development during adolescence.

How much do we grow?

One of the most noticeable features of physical development during infancy and childhood is that we grow taller. There are periods when we experience 'growth spurts' and grow taller, and periods where we tend to develop other physical features such as muscle mass.

1 Look at the following information about an individual's growth from infancy to adulthood.

Age	height gained per year (cm)
0–1	22.5
1–2	20.0
2–3	17.5
3–4	9.0
4–5	7.5
5–6	7.5
6–7	7.0
7–8	7.0
8–9	6.0
9–10	6.0
10–11	5.0
11–12	5.0
12–13	8.0
13–14	8.0
14–15	12.5
15–16	12.5

2 Using the figures above, produce a graph showing the person's growth pattern from birth to the age of 16.

3 Write a paragraph explaining what the figures tell you about the person's pattern of growth.

Build Your Learning

LEARNING POINTS

The following are the main points that you should have learnt from the previous seven pages.

- Human growth and development is a lifelong process.
- Different kinds of change and development occur in each of the various life stages.
- There is an expected, or normal, pattern and sequence of physical growth and developmental change.
- Growth and development is influenced by a range of biological and social factors.

KEY TERMS

You should know what the following terms mean:

- Life stage (page 152)
- Life span (page 152)
- Growth (page 153)
- Development (page 153)
- Developmental norms (page 153)
- Ageing process (page 154)
- Maturation (page 155)

If you're not sure or want to check your understanding, turn to the page number listed in the brackets.

REVISION QUESTIONS

If you're confident that you understand the learning points and the key terms, try answering the revision questions below:

1 What is the difference between:

(a) human growth and human development?

(b) a life stage and a life span?

2 Explain the part that maturation plays in human growth and development.

3 Describe factors that influence emotional development.

The key question that you should be able to answer if you've understood the previous section is:

4 How do individuals grow and develop during each life stage?

INVESTIGATION IDEAS

1 Have a look through your family photographs and identify the ways in which you and your family have changed physically as a result of 'maturation'.

2 Use your school, college or local library to find out more about the work of Jean Piaget. Child development and psychology books are good places to begin looking. Produce a profile and brief notes summarising his ideas on intellectual development.

The first human life stage, from birth to three years, is **infancy**. In the following case study we consider how one person, called Danny James, experienced growth and development as an infant.

CASE STUDY

Danny James is a 3-year-old boy, born and brought up in London. He lives with his parents, and his older sister. Danny currently goes to a playgroup twice a week at the local community centre.

Physical development

Immediately after he was born, and then five minutes later, the midwife checked Danny's physical condition using the Apgar score method (see below). Danny was born with a number of basic physical reflexes (see opposite). For example, as soon as he was born he could breathe, blink his eyes, distinguish colours and smells and suck when something was pushed into his mouth.

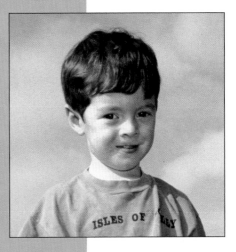

During infancy Danny grew very rapidly. By one year old, he weighed three times his birth weight, was one and a half times as tall, and had a more solid physical frame than when he was born. He also developed some basic movement skills during his first year of life. At first Danny couldn't even hold his head up or reach out for things close to him. In the first few weeks and months of life he developed basic forms of movement, such as holding his head up and moving his arms and legs about. During his first year, Danny was gradually able to hold his head up for longer periods of time, started to reach out for things he could see, and began to crawl.

Observation	Score given		
	0	**1**	**2**
Heart rate	absent	<100/min	<100/min
Respiratory rate	No breathing	Weak cry and shallow breathing	Strong cry and regular breathing
Muscle tone	Flaccid	Some flexion of extremities	Well flexed
Response to stimulation	None	Some motion of feet	Cry
Colour	'Blue'; poor	Body O.K. extremities 'blue'	Good colour all over

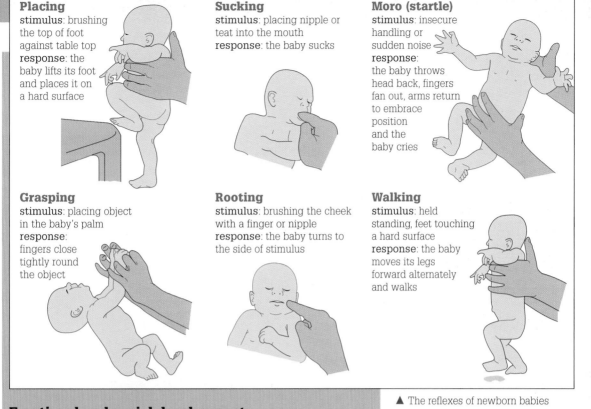

Placing
stimulus: brushing the top of foot against table top
response: the baby lifts its foot and places it on a hard surface

Sucking
stimulus: placing nipple or teat into the mouth
response: the baby sucks

Moro (startle)
stimulus: insecure handling or sudden noise
response: the baby throws head back, fingers fan out, arms return to embrace position and the baby cries

Grasping
stimulus: placing object in the baby's palm
response: fingers close tightly round the object

Rooting
stimulus: brushing the cheek with a finger or nipple
response: the baby turns to the side of stimulus

Walking
stimulus: held standing, feet touching a hard surface
response: the baby moves its legs forward alternately and walks

▲ The reflexes of newborn babies

Emotional and social development

In his first year, Danny had a small circle of people to whom he was emotionally attached. His parents, sister and grandmother were the people who cared for him and with whom he spent most of his time. These people provided Danny with the basic security and safety from which he was able to explore the world around him. By the age of six months, Danny had formed a very strong bond with his mum and dad. Danny, like most babies, became very distressed when he was separated from his parents.

Intellectual development

In common with many other parents, Danny's mum and dad were surprised and excited both by the speed and the ways in which Danny learnt new things. At birth, Danny was able to respond to light and sound in a very simple way. Danny's mum said that he could recognise her face, and smiled at her, when he was just three months old. His dad can remember how Danny gradually made more noise, especially when he was wet or hungry, and could say 'dada' by the time he was nine months old.

Danny's parents said that he was a very curious child, always keen to touch and play with toys, especially those that made a noise! By the age of one, Danny had learnt to recognise his own name and responded to simple words, for example 'good', 'no' and 'well done'. He was gradually learning new words. His first words after 'dada' and 'mama' were 'dog' and 'car'. In his second and third year, Danny's use of language improved a great deal. By the age of three, Danny could hold a simple conversation with any member of his family and had developed a habit of asking lots of questions!

Quick Questions

1 Name two abilities that Danny had when he was born.

2 Describe Danny's growth pattern during his first year.

3 Who helped Danny to develop emotionally during infancy?

4 Name one way Danny developed intellectually during his first year.

In the previous section you learnt about Danny James's physical growth and personal development during infancy. Danny's pattern of growth and development is typical of other children during infancy. In this section we look at the reasons why these changes occur.

Physical growth and development

Physical growth is very rapid and significant during infancy. The physical changes that children experience during this stage of their life transform their appearance and provide a basis for the intellectual, social and emotional development that also occurs. Physical change during infancy is the result of a number of influences.

Influences on growth

Danny's physical growth during infancy was influenced by a number of biological factors. For example, the human body is 'programmed' to mature naturally. Because of this Danny, in common with all babies, moved through a sequence of physical growth and development changes. The genes he inherited from his parents, also influenced Danny's growth pattern and development of physical features.

Danny's pattern of growth and development during this life stage was also influenced by non-biological factors. For example, Danny's parents influenced his physical growth and development by giving him plenty of opportunities to use and develop his body and physical skills through play and other physical activities.

Patterns of development

The changes in physical appearance and ability that Danny experienced in the early months of his life unfolded in a predictable pattern. Physical change in very young infants occurs from the head downwards and from the middle of the body outwards (see opposite). This is the same for all babies who follow developmental norms.

Danny's physical development clearly followed this pattern. For example, he was able to hold his head up without help before he could use his body to sit up. After this he was able to use his legs to crawl. During infancy Danny's bones gradually grew and hardened, and his muscles grew stronger – in the same head-downwards, middle-outwards pattern. This enabled him to carry out new sorts of movement as his body underwent physical development and change.

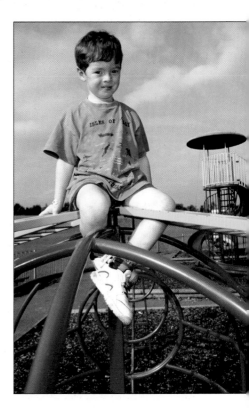

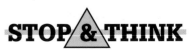

STOP & THINK

What other factors, apart from play, can you think of that may affect a baby's physical growth and development?

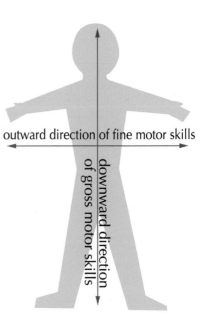

outward direction of fine motor skills

downward direction of gross motor skills

Measuring physical change

It is possible to check whether a child's physical development is within the normal range of what is expected. Centile charts are commonly used to compare a child's pattern of growth to the average growth rates of children of the same age. **Centile charts** of weight and height have been compiled after studying and recording the growth patterns of thousands of children to work out both average and expected patterns. There are different charts for girls and boys. When they are filled in for a specific child, centile charts present clear, visual information about growth.

The bold line on the chart shown opposite represents the average measure of growth in weight expected in male babies over the first 12 months of their life. This means that if a 5-month-old boy weighs 7.8 kg, on average 50 per cent of boys of the same age will weigh less than him and 50 per cent of boys of the same age will weigh more than him. If a boy weighs 13.2 kg at 12 months, then the graph says that 97 per cent of boys of the same age will weigh less than he does and 3 per cent will, on average, weigh more.

By recording a child's growth on centile charts, care workers such as health visitors and GPs can monitor progress and note whether growth is proceeding in an expected pattern.

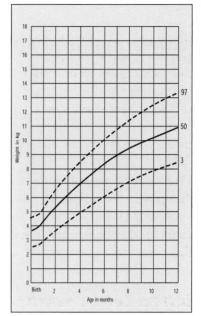

▲ A centile chart for a baby boy

OVER TO YOU

Talk to a parent who has a child under the age of 5 years. Ask him or her to identify the age at which the child first carried out each of the following actions.

- Smiled
- Said his or her first word
- Said his or her first sentence
- Was able to remember and say his or her own name
- Slept through the night without waking
- Was dry throughout the night
- Was dry throughout the day

- Walked without help
- Crawled
- Sat up without support
- Jumped without falling over
- Showed a preference for using one hand or the other
- Built a tower of three bricks
- Began to understand sharing

Find out whether the parent believes that his or her child achieved anything unusually early or later than might be expected. Check this against the expected time for achieving this action and decide whether the parent is correct or not.

Quick Questions

1 Identify two physical factors that influenced Danny's growth and development during infancy.

2 How old was Danny when he first started to crawl?

3 Explain how an infant's growth and development is monitored.

Emotional and social development

An individual's early emotional and social development plays an important part in their future relationships with others. Ideally, children such as Danny James should develop feelings of trust and security early on in their lives. The process through which this occurs is known as **attachment**. Attachment is when a child develops a strong emotional link with his or her parents, or main caregivers. The parental response to this emotional linking is known as **bonding**. Attachment and bonding provide the emotional link between baby and adult through which a first relationship is built.

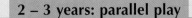

▼ Stages of play

0 – 1 year: solo play

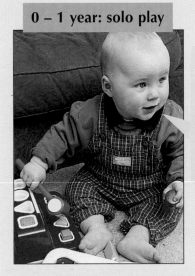

Its difficult for me to think of people other than myself so I like to play on my own. I learn through exploring everything around me.

2 – 3 years: parallel play

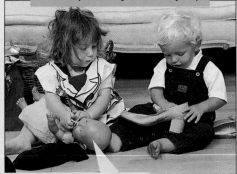

I'm still mainly interested in myself and I can't see the sense of sharing yet. I am interested in other people so I like to be near them. I learn by imitating other people.

3 years old: associative play

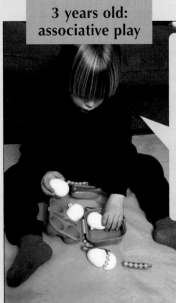

I'm beginning to understand how they feel and to be sympathetic, so that makes it easier to play with other children. I learn a lot by imitating and pretending to be people who are important to me.

over 3 years old: cooperative play

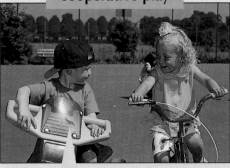

I can see that its more important to share and help other children. I realise that if I cooperate with the other children we have more fun and do more interesting things.

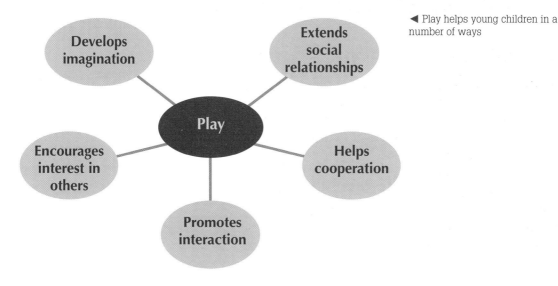

◀ Play helps young children in a number of ways

Four things influence the quality of the bond:

■ how sensitively the mother understands and responds to the baby's needs

■ the personality of the mother

■ the consistency of the care that the baby receives

■ the baby's own temperament.

Emotional and social development during infancy is extremely important. It is thought that a person's earliest relationships provide a 'blueprint' or model for the relationships that they develop in later life. Like Danny, children tend gradually to increase their social relationships by including brothers, sisters, relatives and perhaps neighbours' children in their social circle. The nature of the social contacts that children have at this stage is influenced by their emerging **communication skills**. As they progress through infancy, children are increasingly able to look at the world from the point of view of other people. This is demonstrated by the gradual changes in the way in which children in this age group (like Danny) play (see opposite).

Successful social relationships among children are helped by:

■ secure attachment in their early years

■ opportunities to mix with other children, especially where they involve activities that require co-operation

■ the personality of the child: children who are friendly, supportive and optimistic make friends more easily than children who are negative and aggressive.

Quick Questions

1 Identify the emotional qualities that a child develops through a close attachment to a parent or carer.

2 Describe the kinds of factors that help children to develop successful social relationships.

3 Explain why early relationships are thought to play an important part in a person's emotional development when they are older.

Intellectual development

Intellectual development involves changes in a person's thinking, memory and language ability. Changes begin as soon as a person is born and never really end until death. Infancy is a life stage when a great deal of basic intellectual development takes place.

Influences on intellectual development

Intellectual development during infancy is mainly a matter of maturing. It is generally thought that infants are born with the capacity to learn, think and use language. The environment in which an infant lives is thought to influence the speed and extent to which he or she develops these skills. Intellectual ability during this life stage is therefore said to be a matter of both nature and nurture.

As an infant, Danny James saw and experienced many things that were new to him. Danny, in common with most children, used these new experiences to acquire quickly a better understanding of the world around him. This type of early learning happens continuously and is very important for young children.

Stages of development

Jean Piaget, a psychologist, identified a number of stages of intellectual development, with the first beginning in infancy. He saw infancy as the time when children went through what he called the **sensorimotor stage** of intellectual development. This stage is said to occur between birth and two years of age. During this stage, babies learn a lot about themselves and the world around them through their senses (touch, hearing, sight, smell, and taste – hence 'sensori') and through physical activity (also known as motor activity). A very important lesson that children learn during this stage is that objects and people in the world continue to exist even when they can't be seen. This might seem obvious to you now, but it's not to a young baby. In early infancy, before eight months old, children won't usually search for an object that's hidden. To them, it no longer seems to exist. In later infancy they will search, as they develop what is known as **object permanence**. In other words, they learn that objects do still exist even though they can't be seen.

Language development

A second key feature of intellectual development during infancy is learning the basics of a spoken language. Caregivers responsible for young children have an important role to play in helping children to communicate effectively and to use language in a wide variety of ways. While children do not actually use their first proper words until they are about a year old, babies begin developing communication skills almost straight from birth.

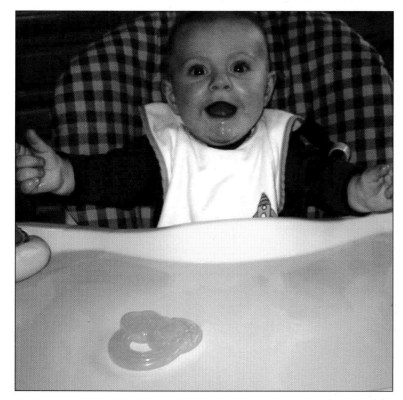

◄ Young babies can communicate a lot of things without using any words at all

The initial communications of babies are in the form of smiles, movements and noises that are part of a 'conversation' with a caregiver. The baby is already able to give and receive information and to communicate feelings. Young children move rapidly through the different stages of language development, from babbling (between eight to ten months old), to their first words (between a year and two years of age), to short sentences (from about 18 months old). By two and half years, children are learning a few new words a day, so that by the age of three they have a vocabulary of about a thousand words.

Although children can talk effectively by the time they are three years old, it is not correct to think that language development ends there. Language learning continues throughout childhood and people continue to refine their use of language throughout life.

Quick Questions

1 Identify the kinds of changes that an infant experiences as a result of intellectual development.

2 Describe how children learn new things during the sensorimotor stage of development.

3 Explain what would happen (and why) if you hid a toy that a one-year-old child was playing with

The second life stage is childhood (from four to ten years old). In the following case study we consider how Rachel James is developing.

CASE STUDY

Rachel James is Danny's older sister. She attends primary school where she has many friends. Rachel is learning to swim and is looking forward to going to the seaside for a summer holiday.

Physical growth and development

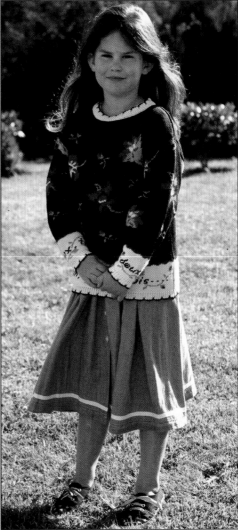

Between the ages of four and six years, Rachel learnt to run, jump, hop and ride a bicycle. She enjoys playing ball games and skipping and is now a very active, energetic child. Rachel's physical appearance has changed a lot during the last few years. As she's lost her baby fat she's become less top-heavy than she was as an infant, and has become more physically co-ordinated. She is also stronger, and able to move in more subtle and sophisticated ways.

During the next few years Rachel's muscle tissue will increase and she will become taller, stronger and more robust. She will develop much more distinct physical features than in the previous phase. By her late childhood, Rachel will have developed facial features that will change very little throughout her adult life. Her physical growth will progress slowly and gradually in this phase until puberty begins in about her twelfth year.

Social and emotional development

During her early childhood Rachel has faced a number of social and emotional challenges. The birth of her brother Danny was an important event. Rachel developed a close relationship with Danny. However, she also had to learn cope with being part of a bigger family where Danny also needed time and attention from her parents. Going to school was the next major event in Rachel's life. It meant being with other children, making new friendships and listening to people who were not her parents or close family members. Rachel found this difficult at first but now enjoys going to school. In this stage of her childhood Rachel began to acquire new communication skills (language and listening) and social behaviours and used these to build relationships with a broad range of people, including new friends and school staff. Rachel's social world expanded rapidly after she started going to school.

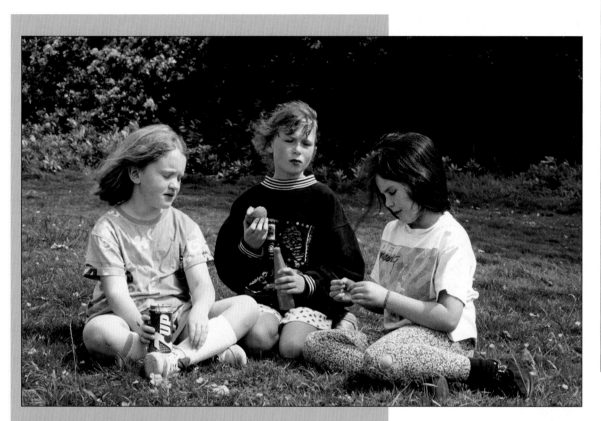

Intellectual development

In her first year at primary school Rachel began to organise her thinking more. She was keen to learn new things and participate in class activities. Rachel's speech quickly became more sophisticated as she learnt more words and improved her ways of using them. At school Rachel learnt how to read and write and developed the ability to think about, and work out her own solutions to, simple problems and the frustrations that she faced.

Rachel's knowledge, vocabulary and learning skills have expanded dramatically since she started school in her early childhood. The knowledge and abilities that she has developed are used in all areas of her life, both in and out of school. For example, Rachel is now very interested in going to a Brownie group, and in taking part in her local swimming club. She's using and expanding her intellectual, physical and social skills in both these out-of-school clubs.

Quick Questions

1 Name one way in which a child like Rachel has developed (not grown!) physically since infancy.

2 Describe two ways in which children use social skills to adapt to life outside their family home.

3 Explain how going to school may have helped Rachel's development.

Physical growth and development

Have you been to a primary school recently? If so, you might have noticed that learning activities in the reception and early infants classes are often directed towards refining and expanding the co-ordination and fine motor skills that young children begin to develop at this stage in their lives. Rachel was able to do many of the physical activities described in the case study because she passed rapidly through the stage of physical development where her balance control improved.

Social and emotional development

During early childhood children like Danny and Rachel need to develop relationships with children and adults outside their own family. It is at this time that children first leave their parents to go to school. This broadens their relationships and expands their social world, but it can be emotionally difficult. You may still remember how you felt when your parents left you at the school gate on your first day at school and went home without you! The first days at primary school are very distressing for some children.

During this life stage, children have to learn to co-operate, communicate and spend time with a new set of adults and children. Most children gradually increase their self-confidence and independence during this stage. A variety of nature and nurture factors influence the extent to which individual children develop their personal confidence and independence. For example, a child who feels encouraged and supported and who has good role models develops his or her self-confidence and sense of independence more easily than a child who is criticised, discouraged and over-protected during his or her early childhood.

Intellectual development

The second stage of intellectual development in Piaget's theory (see page 157 and 166) is called the **pre-operational stage**. This is said to occur between the ages of two and seven years. In this stage, children like Rachel James are less reliant on physical learning (seeing, touching and holding things) because they develop the ability to think about objects that are not actually there in front of them. Nevertheless, children's thinking in this life stage is still limited. They still tend to think about everything from their own point of view and are not aware that others may have different viewpoints. This is known as **egocentrism**.

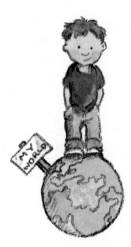

Rachel's knowledge, vocabulary and learning skills have expanded dramatically since she started school in her early childhood. The knowledge and abilities that she has developed are used in all areas of her life, both in and out of school. For example, Rachel is now very interested in going to a Brownie group, and in taking part in her local swimming club. She's using and expanding her intellectual, physical and social skills in both these out-of-school clubs.

Moral development

During early childhood an important change occurs in a child's sense of values and in the way that they think. A child's **conscience** – the ability to decide what is good or bad and to distinguish between right and wrong in his or her own and other people's behaviour – is said to develop through three stages.

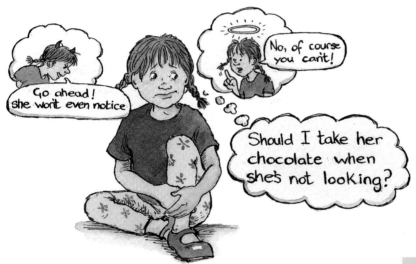

At first, children tend to base their judgements about right and wrong on the rules they have been taught by the people in their lives with authority, such as parents and teachers. Then, during early childhood, children usually conform to rules if doing so means that they will avoid being punished or that they will receive rewards. The standards of morality that are taught or demonstrated by parents tend to have a big influence on young children who wish to be a 'good boy' or 'good girl'. This lasts until they reach adolescence. In the final phase of development, during adolescence, making moral judgements becomes a more sophisticated process (see page 175 for more details about this).

Quick Questions

1 Name some of the environmental factors that are said to stimulate social development during childhood.

2 Describe how a child's self-confidence and independence can be nurtured.

3 Young children are said to be egocentric. Explain what this term means.

The third life stage is **adolescence** (11–18 years). The following case study describes how Rachel James will develop into an adolescent (teenager).

CASE STUDY

Rachel James is now eight years old and settled at school. She will experience puberty in the next four or five years.

Physical growth and development

When Rachel enters puberty she is likely to experience a 'growth spurt'. This means that her body will grow and change very rapidly. Rachel's puberty will also involve the development of **secondary sexual characteristics**. This will begin with the growth of pubic hair and Rachel's breasts will begin to develop. She will also experience further growth of her uterus and vagina, widening of her hips and the onset of her menstrual cycle.

In common with most boys, Danny James is not likely to experience an adolescent growth spurt and significant physical change until he reaches the age of 13. When this happens, the first indication of puberty is likely to be the growth of his testes, scrotum and pubic hair. Danny will grow body hair (on his face and chest and in his armpits) and his voice will get deeper. Danny will grow to his maximum height and develop greater muscle bulk.

Emotional and social development

When Rachel begins to progress through adolescence she will experience a period of major emotional change and social development. When she reaches adulthood, her parents, like those of many other people, will probably look back and say that they had most problems with her during this life stage!

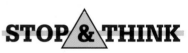

STOP & THINK

Why do you think parents often find their teenage children difficult to cope with?

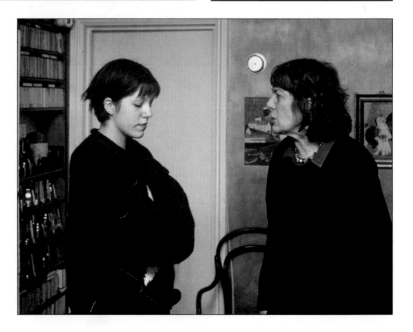

▶ Emotions and relationships can feel intense and be difficult for many adolescents to manage.

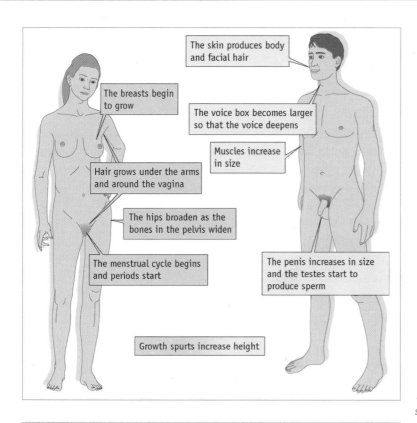

The skin produces body and facial hair

The breasts begin to grow

The voice box becomes larger so that the voice deepens

Muscles increase in size

Hair grows under the arms and around the vagina

The hips broaden as the bones in the pelvis widen

The menstrual cycle begins and periods start

The penis increases in size and the testes start to produce sperm

Growth spurts increase height

◀ The development of secondary sexual characteristics

Rachel will expand her social circle, and her friends or **peer group** will become more important to her. She will try to break free from the authority of her parents and seek to be much more independent. In common with most adolescent girls, Rachel will begin to look for a partner. Experimenting with intimate relationships, whether they involve sexual activity or not, will lead Rachel to experience the positive and negative emotions that can result from close relationships. Socially and emotionally, adolescence is likely to be an exciting and at times difficult life stage for Rachel. Her search for identity and independence will sometimes bring her into conflict with her parents, teachers and friends. It should also lead her to achieve greater self-confidence and a sense of who she is, the sorts of friends she prefers and the kind of partner she is seeking.

Intellectual development

Rachel will attend secondary school and take public examinations, such as GCSEs, during adolescence. She will learn many new skills, develop her knowledge of different subjects and be required to remember and think about a huge amount of information during this time. The way that Rachel thinks will change from the way that she thought during childhood. She is likely to develop the ability to use abstract thinking and may doubt, and rebel against, her parents' ideas of what is good and bad, right and wrong. Intellectual development during adolescence will enable Rachel to question what she is told and she will begin to develop a sense of her own values.

Quick Questions

1 Identify three physical changes that girls experience during puberty.

2 Describe one likely consequence on the relationship she has with her parents of Rachel's intellectual development during adolescence.

3 Explain what the term 'peer group' means.

Adolescence begins at about the age of 11 years and ends somewhere between 16 and 22. This stage of maturation is called **puberty**. In terms of physical growth and change, and emotional, social and intellectual development, adolescence is a very active phase.

You will have noticed in the case study about the adolescent life stage that we described how Rachel and Danny James would grow and develop in the future. It is possible to do this because individual development follows a relatively predictable pattern. You might remember that we called this 'normal development' earlier in this unit (see page 153). One stage of development that most readers of this book will have recent experience of is adolescence. We will now look at the growth and development changes that occur during puberty.

Physical growth and change

The growth spurt and physical changes that occur in puberty are caused by an increase in the activity of **hormones**. Hormones are chemical secretions that pass directly into the blood from the endocrine glands.

The two main glands that secrete the hormones affecting growth and development are the thyroid gland and the pituitary gland. Several different hormones are secreted by each of these glands (see opposite).

The pituitary gland is located at the base of the brain. It is only about the size of a pea, but is nevertheless very important in controlling the hormone production affecting growth and development.

The thyroid gland is located in the neck. It also has an important influence on general growth rate, bone and muscle development and in the function of the reproductive organs. During puberty, the testes (in boys) produce the hormone testosterone and the ovaries (in girls) produce oestrogen and progesterone. These hormones control the development and function of the reproductive organs.

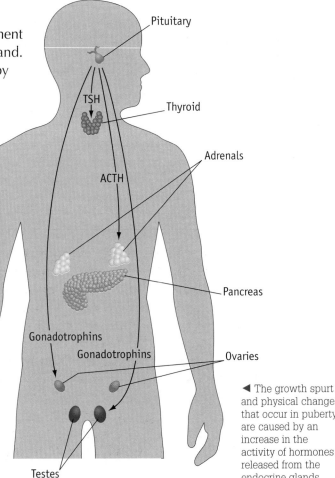

◀ The growth spurt and physical changes that occur in puberty are caused by an increase in the activity of hormones released from the endocrine glands

Emotional and social development

In terms of social and emotional development, puberty and adolescence can be both a difficult and a very active time. The need for an individual identity and a sense of social and emotional belonging are important concerns in this phase. Adolescents usually experiment with intimate personal relationships with members of the opposite sex, and sometimes the same sex, as they explore their sexuality and the positive and negative emotions that result from close relationships. This experimentation may include making decisions about whether or not to engage in sexual activity as part of an intimate personal relationship. In this phase of social and emotional development, individuals tend to gain greater understanding of the thoughts, feelings and motives of others.

Intellectual development

Intellectual development during adolescence mainly involves the emergence of abstract thinking. A person who can think abstractly can think about things that aren't actually there and things that don't actually exist. This sounds a bit odd but it is probably a feature of your own thinking that you now take for granted. For example, algebraic equations involve abstract thinking, as does thinking about the beginning of the universe. However, a more enjoyable way of testing whether you can think abstractly might be imagining what it would be like to be stranded on a tropical island with your favourite film, or television, star! Abstract thinking is considered to be the final stage of thought development. Intellectual development is not completed in adolescence however, but continues throughout life.

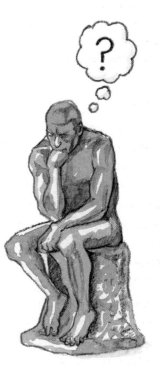

Moral development

The way people think about moral issues, such as right and wrong, changes during adolescence. During adolescence, individuals typically base their judgements about right and wrong on the rules, or **norms**, of the social groups to which they belong. These include family, friendship and peer groups, church groups and clubs. However, whereas children believe that good behaviour is whatever pleases important individuals in their lives, adolescents tend to be guided by the more abstract laws and rules of society. Adolescents are more likely to be guided by a sense of duty to conform to the general rules of their social groups rather than obeying the specific things their parents tell them. Being law abiding and a good citizen is more important than being a good boy or girl.

Quick Questions

1 Name the new type of thinking ability that many adolescents develop.

2 Describe the effects of two factors that affect growth and development during puberty. You should choose one nature factor and one nurture factor.

3 What reasons can you give to explain why individuals come into conflict with their parents more during adolescence than in childhood?

Normally, the longest life stage is adulthood (19 years old to 65 years old). The latter part of adulthood is often referred to as middle age. The following case study looks at Danny and Rachel James' parents, Tom and Laura.

CASE STUDY

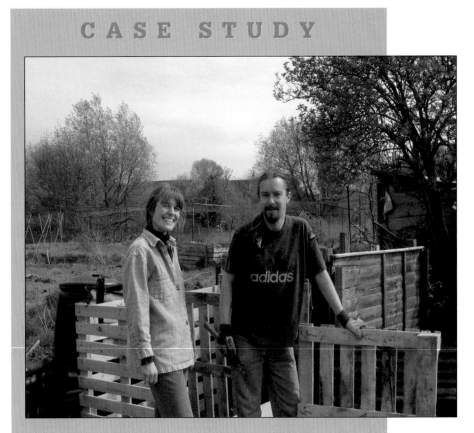

Tom and Laura James have been married for eight years. Both were born and brought up in Manchester. Tom and Laura came to live in London six years ago. Tom is a social worker with a local authority. Laura works part time as a primary school teacher.

Physical growth and development

Physically, both Tom and Laura are in the prime of their lives. At 30 years old, Laura is in the first half of early adulthood. Tom at 35 years old is in the second half of early adulthood. Laura and Tom have produced two children and can have more children, until Laura experiences the menopause in later adulthood. They would like one more child to complete their family.

Tom and Laura are fit and healthy at this point in their lives. Laura is a keen swimmer and says that her strength, speed and stamina when swimming are the best they've ever been. Tom likes to go jogging but says that he is no longer as fast, or as light, as he once was. Tom has recently started to lose some of his hair and predicts that he will go bald, like his father, by the time he is 50 years old!

Emotional and social development

Developing a close intimate relationship, getting married and having children has fundamentally altered Laura's and Tom's lives over the last eight years. They are very committed to their role as parents, though both are also keen to develop their careers and currently enjoy their jobs. Work, children and marriage will be the key influences on Laura's and Tom's social and emotional development during adulthood. Their circle of friends, ambitions and emotional life are all likely to be focused on raising their family successfully, succeeding at work and developing their relationship.

Intellectual development

Laura is a qualified primary school teacher and Tom is a qualified social worker. Both are continuing to develop their careers by taking courses and learning about new developments in their fields of work. In their leisure time Laura and Tom both enjoy reading, watching films, going to museums and travelling abroad on holidays. At this stage in their lives, Laura and Tom are learning many new things and are using their intellectual abilities and experience in their everyday lives.

Family life and work seem to be the most important things in both our lives at the moment. Life changed a lot when the children were born. Suddenly we had much less time for ourselves – and we always have to plan our free time around the needs of the children! But things are always changing, aren't they? I'm not saying we've got no time for each other. We've got lots to look forward to, and our personal lives haven't stopped. They've just got more complicated!

Quick Questions

1 Which life stage are Tom and Laura currently in?
2 Describe the key events that have affected Tom's and Laura's emotional development since they married.
3 Explain the role that friendships play in social development during adulthood.

Adulthood is the life stage that people commonly think of as being 'grown up'. If you look back at the diagram of the development process, on page 153, you will see that adulthood is, in some ways, the high point of human development. It is the developmental stage at which people have achieved their maximum physical size and capacity and the stage at which their intellectual abilities are at their peak. We will now look at the different features of adult growth and development described in the case study.

Physical growth and development

Physical changes in adulthood are not like the changes that occur in childhood and adolescence – they are not about improvement. Growth is largely complete by the end of adolescence. By the time a person reaches adulthood he or she is grown up. People in their early twenties to early thirties are capable of achieving their maximum physical performance. You may have noticed that most athletes and sports professionals achieve their best performances while they are young adults.

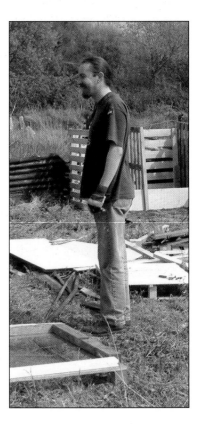

In the second half of this phase, from about 30 years to 42 years adults, like Tom who is 35 years old, experience an increase in the amount of fatty tissue in their bodies, move more slowly and take longer to recover from their efforts. Men may also start to lose their hair or go grey and women start to get wrinkles around their eyes as their skin becomes less supple.

When Tom and Laura reach the middle of their life span, sometime from their forties to late fifties, they will undergo many physical changes. During this later phase of adulthood many people experience diminishing abilities and a decline in physical performance compared to earlier stages of their life. The physical changes that human beings experience during adulthood and older age are often referred to as **ageing**. The physical effects of the ageing process can be most clearly seen by contrasting the physical condition, appearance and abilities of a person during early adulthood with those in old age.

The role of hormones

During late adulthood, both men and women experience the loss of their ability to reproduce. In men this occurs gradually as their levels of testosterone gradually decline throughout adulthood. A better-known physical change is the one affecting women. **Menopause**, or the ending of menstruation and the ability to produce children, occurs because a woman's ovaries produce less and less of the hormones oestrogen and progesterone until a point is reached at which the ovaries stop producing eggs.

Emotional and social development

It is difficult to generalise about what happens in terms of social and emotional development in this phase, because of the huge diversity of experience among people. During adulthood people may experience a number of transitions with emotional and social consequences. Marriage and divorce, parenthood and increasing work responsibility, and the loss of elderly parents are all life events most likely to be experienced during adulthood. This life stage tends to revolve around people trying to achieve their position in society and their ambitions in life.

Intellectual development

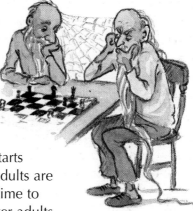

As adults, Tom and Laura James are capable of abstract thought, have memories functioning at their peak and can think very quickly. However, compared to older adults, people in this phase lack experience of the world. In contrast, in later adulthood the capacity for quick, reactive thought begins to diminish and memory starts to become slower. This does not mean that older adults are any less capable, just that they may require more time to perform the same intellectual activities than younger adults do. Because older people have a greater breadth and depth of knowledge, gained from experience, they tend to use this to be more analytical and reflective in their thinking

Moral development

During adulthood some individuals find that they need to revise their ways of judging right and wrong and making other moral judgements. This happens when people discover that the social rules and laws, which they followed in adolescence, are inadequate. Life is often just too complex for simple, clear-cut rules. Some adults develop what is known as **principled morality**. This means they tend to make judgements on self-chosen principles. They discover situations where they feel that rules and laws need to be ignored or changed and try to use universal principles such as truth, equality and social justice to make their decisions. This way of thinking about moral issues is clearly very different from that of children who apply simple rules to gain approval from parents and other people.

Quick Questions

1 What development-related reasons can you give to explain why most athletics records are set by people in early adulthood?

2 What features of ageing begin to emerge in men and women from mid-adulthood onwards?

3 Explain what happens during menopause.

4 Identify a number of factors that affect emotional and social development during adulthood.

5 Can an individual's judgement of moral issues develop further during adulthood?

The final life stage, 65 years and over, is illustrated in the following case study about Tom's mother, Audrey.

CASE STUDY

Tom's mother, Audrey James, is 73 years of age. She still lives in Manchester and shares a house with one of her other sons and his family.

Physical change

Audrey has experienced a number of changes in her appearance and physical functioning over the last twenty years of her life. She experienced the menopause in her mid fifties and began hormone replacement therapy to counter some of the effects of this.

Audrey has been in relatively good physical health in the last few years, though she has noticed more aches and pains, and sometimes complains of stiffness in her ankle and elbow joints. Over the last ten years Audrey's skin has become noticeably more wrinkled.

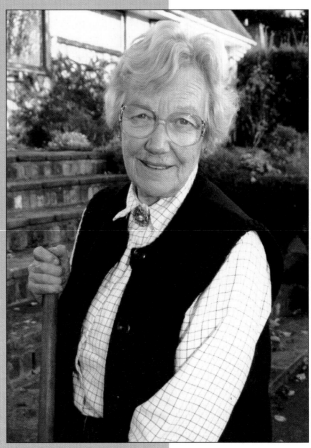

Her hair went grey in her early fifties and then turned white a few years ago. Audrey's GP (family doctor) has told her that she's also experienced a slight decrease in height in the last few years. Despite these physical changes, Audrey is still a very active person. She tends to walk more slowly and has less stamina than she used to have, but compensates for this by taking rests and planning her journeys carefully. Like most other people at this stage of life, Audrey has also experienced sensory changes as her hearing and sight have deteriorated.

Emotional and social development

Audrey's personal and family relationships have changed a lot over the past few years. Her husband, Harry, died last year and had been ill for two years before that. Since his death, Audrey has become very close to her son, daughter-in-law and their children. She has a very strong sense of being a part of a caring family and now feels very emotionally attached to her children and grandchildren. Audrey is very proud of all her grandchildren as well as her own children and their partners. Her social relationships with friends and other people outside the immediate family are still important to her, though she tends to see less and less of the friends who were part of her earlier adult life with Harry. Audrey is quite reflective when she talks with her family members and friends who visit her at home – reviewing her achievements and her relationships.

Intellectual change and development

Audrey has always been interested in solving puzzles and problems. She worked for a firm of accountants as a bookkeeper before she got married, and returned to this when her children were at school. Audrey now enjoys reading, watches a lot of films on television and plays chess and other board games as a hobby. She often attends a local community centre where she meets up with some of her friends. They spend the afternoon chatting, playing games and occasionally listening to invited speakers or taking part in dance or exercise classes.

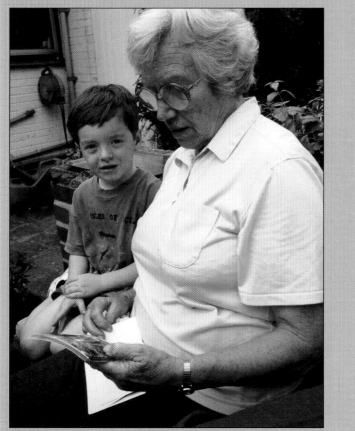

Audrey uses her bookkeeping knowledge to help the parents running the nursery that one of her grandchildren attends. She also takes him to the nursery and does the accounts when required. Audrey enjoys reading stories and singing nursery rhymes with the children.

Quick Questions

1 Identify three physical aspects of the ageing process that Audrey has experienced.

2 Describe how Audrey may have been affected emotionally by the death of her husband.

3 Explain how Audrey tries to maintain her intellectual development.

The process of physical ageing quickens for all people from about the age of 55 years. By the age of 75 years the physical effects of ageing are clearly evident. Later adulthood, also known as old age, is a time of diminishing physical capabilities and changing emotional experiences, intellectual interests and social circumstances. Ageing inevitably involves physical change but this doesn't mean that when people reach old age they suddenly become unwell, infirm or in need of care. Many older people are physically healthy and robust.

Ageing is a gradual process that is most recognisable in the physical differences that can be seen between people in adulthood and old age. Less visible social, emotional and intellectual changes also occur during this period. While many, usually young people, view old age in a negative way, the gradual decline in abilities that occurs doesn't necessarily mean that older people have a poor quality of life or are unhappy.

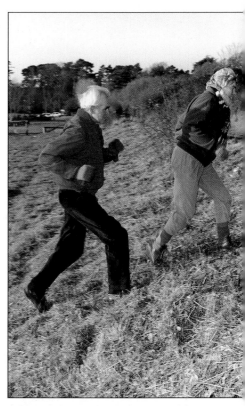

▲ Many older people enjoy an active life

Physical change

During old age, people experience physical decline with poorer heart and lung function, muscle wastage, brittle bones and stiff joints. These changes are part of the normal ageing process.

- The skin becomes less elastic, losing the thin underlying layer of fat, and becomes drier and more fragile. Skin changes include the eventual development of wrinkles.

- Hair usually changes colour, turning grey and then white, becoming finer and thinner at the same time. Many men, and a smaller proportion of women, lose hair from the top of the head.

- Mental functioning tends to get slower. The speed at which older people are able to think and respond is generally reduced, and they may experience poor short-term memory, but mental capacity and intelligence are not lost. Older people do not become any less intelligent as a result of ageing.

- Hearing tends to deteriorate slowly as people age. Quiet and high-pitched sounds (and voices!) become more difficult to hear.

- Sight is affected as people age because the lens in the eye loses its elasticity. The result is that older people find it harder to focus on close objects.

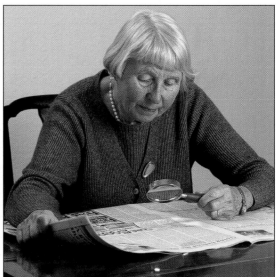

- Weakening of bones, also known as osteoporosis, occurs in old age. Calcium and protein are lost from the bones and older people can become physically frail and experience fractures (broken bones) as a result.

- Posture becomes bent and height is reduced due to thinning of the intervertebral discs with age.

Emotional and social change

Social and emotional development takes on a new importance in the later stages of the life span. Audrey, in common with many older people, must come to terms with the changes in her relationships – her children have grown up, her husband has died and her circle of friends has reduced. Older people continue to develop and change emotionally as they experience new life events and transitions, such as becoming grandparents and retiring from work. They may have more leisure time in which to build relationships with friends and family members. However, older people can experience insecurity and loneliness if retirement or bereavement reduces social contacts.

Intellectual change

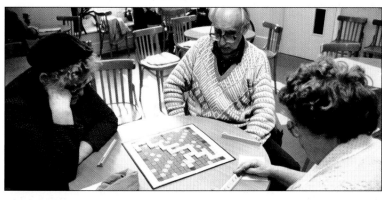

◀ Ageing doesn't necessarily reduce intellectual ability

Older people use and maintain their intellectual abilities in much the same ways as adults and middle-aged people. Both the young-old (60–75 years) and the old-old (75 years and over) need, and enjoy, intellectually stimulating activities in their lives. There are many negative ideas about older people's intellectual abilities. While it is true that a minority of older people develop dementia-related illnesses with memory loss, the majority of older people do not. They can perform the same intellectual activities as younger people, although sometimes a little more slowly. People who develop dementia-related illnesses tend to have memory problems, especially in recalling recently acquired information, and they become confused more easily. These types of illnesses also result in sufferers gradually losing speech and other abilities that are controlled by the brain.

Quick Questions

1 Is it true that people lose some height in old age?

2 Describe the cause and effects of osteoporosis.

3 Which recent event has had a major effect on Audrey's emotional development?

4 What are the key features of dementia-related illness?

5 Explain why people develop wrinkles as they grow older.

We all have a view of the sort of person we are. These views are referred to as our 'self-concept'. As we mature and are influenced by different experiences and our relationships with other people throughout our life cycle, our self-concept develops and changes. At the same time, we are growing and developing physically, socially and intellectually. This activity gives you the opportunity to think about and express your own self-concept and to interview another person about theirs.

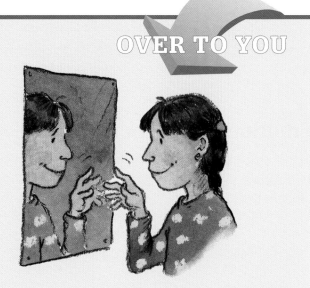

1 For each of the life stages outlined below identify a main feature of growth or development that individuals are likely experience if they follow a pattern of 'normal development'.

Life-stage	Physical	Intellectual	Emotional	Social
Infancy				
Childhood				
Adolescence				
Adulthood				
Mid-life				
Old-age				

Build Your Learning

LEARNING POINTS

The following are the main points that you should have learnt from the previous 25 pages.

- Human growth and development occur in each of the five main human life stages.
- Physical growth is a feature of the first three life stages but is usually complete by adulthood.
- Biological, or nature factors, including hormones and maturation processes, have a considerable influence on the pattern of physical growth.
- Environmental, or nurture factors, such as friendships, education and stimulation, have a considerable effect on the pattern of an individual's intellectual, emotional and social development.

REVISION QUESTIONS

If you're confident that you understand the learning points and the key terms, try answering the revision questions below:

1 Describe the expected pattern of human physical growth between birth and adulthood.

2 Explain the role that environmental factors play in intellectual development throughout the life span.

3 Explain why successful attachment and bonding are seen as vital for an individual's emotional and social development.

The key question that you should be able to answer if you've understood the previous section is:

4 'How do individuals grow and develop during each life stage?'

KEY TERMS

You should know what the following terms mean:

- Infancy (page 160)
- Centile charts (page 163)
- Attachment (page 164)
- Bonding (page 164)
- Sensorimotor stage (page 166)
- Object permanence (page 166)
- Pre-operational stage (page 170)
- Egocentrism (page 170)
- Conscience (page 171)
- Adolescence (page 172)
- Secondary sexual characteristics (page 172)
- Peer group (page 173)
- Puberty (page 174)
- Hormones (page 174)
- Norms (page 175)
- Menopause (page 178)
- Principled morality (page 179)

If you're not sure or want to check your understanding of a term, turn to the page number in the bracket after the word.

INVESTIGATION IDEAS

1 Use your knowledge and understanding of human growth and development to produce a set of questions that you could use to interview an adult or older person about their pattern of growth and development. You need to ensure that your interviewee is a willing volunteer and is happy for you to write about the things they tell you.

2 Talk to your parents about your own early growth and development. Try and find out whether you followed the expected pattern of development, when you reached different 'milestones' and what their memories are of you as a baby and infant.

3 What are the good things about growing older? Talk to an older person, perhaps someone who is a relative or friend, and ask about their thoughts and feelings on growing old. Try to find out about the positive and enjoyable aspects of later adulthood.

What makes human beings grow and develop? In particular, what causes us to change in the various ways that we do? One way of answering this question is to say that people grow and develop through the combined effects of nature and nurture. These two factors are explained in the following pages.

The influence of nature

When people refer to **nature** or natural influences on growth and development they are pointing to the effects that biological, mainly genetic, factors have on human growth and development. The genes we inherit from our parents play a very important role in determining our physical growth and appearance, and also on the abilities we develop.

Each of our body cells contains two sets of 23 chromosomes – one set from each parent.

Each chromosome can contain up to 4,000 different genes. These are the 'instructions' or codes that tell our body's cells how to grow. The genes that determine how we grow as individuals are a unique combination of our biological parents' genes. A consequence of this is that we can do very little to change our physical features and growth potential. We inherit our growth potential from our parents. If both your biological parents are over six-feet tall, have large feet and are fast runners then you are also likely to grow tall, have large feet and be able to run fast. As you grow and develop your genetic inheritance will lead you to look like one or both of your parents as the 'instructions' in your genes are expressed. This is nature at work.

Genes carry masses of information that affects how a person grows and develops. Often a person's genes are responsible for the illnesses and diseases they develop during their lifetime. This is because many people inherit a tendency or predisposition to conditions such as heart disease, cancers and strokes. For example, a person who inherits 'heart disease genes' is more likely to suffer from heart disease than is someone who doesn't inherit these genes. Whether the vulnerable person goes on to develop heart disease or not depends on many factors, especially those related to how they live their life.

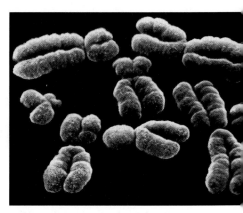

▲ An electron micrograph scan of a group of human chromosomes. Each chromosome is capable of making an exact replica of itself.

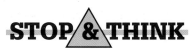

STOP & THINK

How are you physically similar to, and different from, your parents? How can the differences be explained?

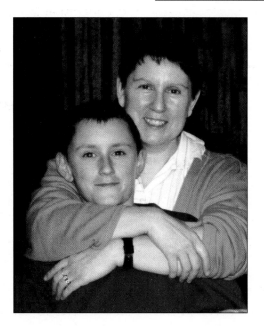

The influence of nurture

Physical growth and change cannot be fully explained by nature alone. Our physical growth is also affected by **nurture.** Nurture includes the many caring and environmental factors that contribute to a person's development. For example, even if both your parents are six feet tall and can run fast, you still might not grow to your full height and develop your running potential if you are malnourished and take no exercise during childhood and adolescence. Good food and exercise are environmental or external influences because they affect a person's growth and development from outside the body. Nature factors (such as genes) are internal influences; they affect growth and development from inside the body.

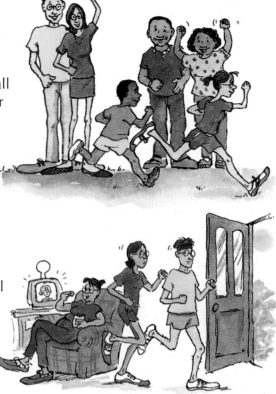

Nurture, or the environment, has a very powerful effect in shaping our social, emotional and intellectual development, as well as some influence on our physical growth. For example, bad housing conditions and not having enough food to eat are environmental factors that often lead to poor growth in children, and illness in people of all ages.

Nature and nurture combined

In reality, a person's growth and development are influenced by both nature and nurture factors. The discussion about which has the more powerful effect is sometimes called the nature-nurture debate. The only safe conclusion in this debate is that people develop through the combined effects of nature and nurture. However, nature cannot be changed. Whereas the ways in which people are nurtured can be controlled and changed.

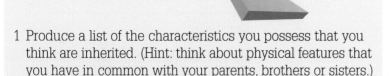

OVER TO YOU

1 Produce a list of the characteristics you possess that you think are inherited. (Hint: think about physical features that you have in common with your parents, brothers or sisters.)

2 Produce a second list of the environmental influences that have played a role in your development. (Hint: think about the important experiences and features of your surroundings that have affected you.)

Quick Questions

1 How many chromosomes are normally contained in each body cell?

2 Explain, in your own words, how genes affect growth and development.

3 Describe how environmental factors can affect a person's growth and development.

We develop our individual social, emotional and intellectual abilities during each life stage. Our gender and ethnicity play an important part in shaping our development in these areas.

Gender

A person's sex is biologically determined. Genes determine whether a person is male or female. Gender, on the other hand, is a socially defined characteristic and plays an important part in social and emotional development. In present-day Western societies girls are taught, or socialised, to take on and express 'feminine' qualities (being kind, caring and gentle, for example) and boys are socialised to express 'masculine' characteristics (such as being boisterous, aggressive and tough). Parents, schools, friends and the media all play a part in socialising, or teaching, children and young people to develop and express the gender qualities associated with their biological sex.

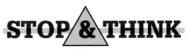

STOP & THINK

How are young children socialised into gender roles? Try and identify ways in which boys and girls are treated differently.

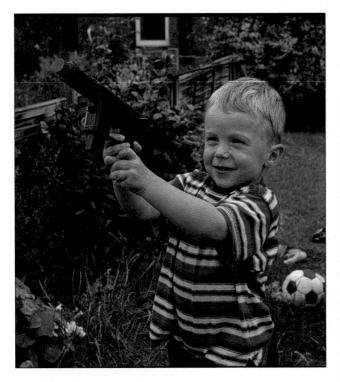

The gender expectations that we experience as we develop influence our personalities and behaviour and affect the ways in which we experience the world and are treated by others.

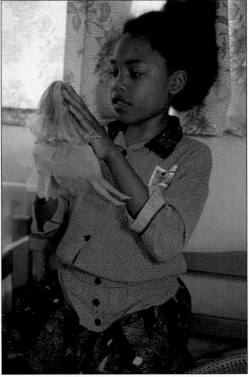

▲ Do toys create or reflect differences in the behaviour of boys and girls?

Ethnicity

Ethnicity, like gender, is socially defined. People tend to define their own ethnicity, and that of other people, according to the characteristics that lead them to belong to a particular community. For example, where people have a shared history or culture, a common geographical origin, a particular skin colour, or a common language or religion, they are seen as having a shared **ethnicity**.

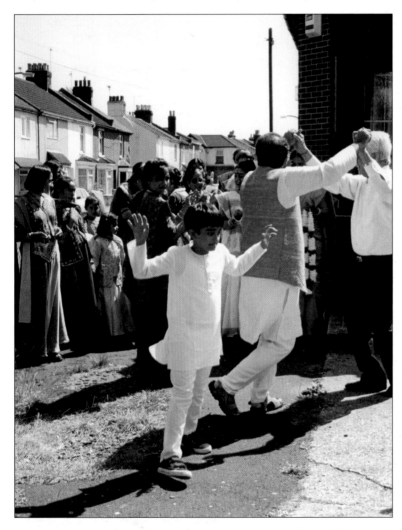

Ethnicity is often an important feature of a person's identity. It may affect personal development because it leads the individual to seek out and take part in particular activities or social groups. It may also be a label (for example, 'Asian', 'Black', 'Welsh') that influences how other people treat and respond to the person. This in itself can have a powerful effect on personal development.

STOP & THINK

How do you and your friends define your ethnicity? Make a list of the factors that play a part in this.

Quick Questions

1 Is gender a result of nature or nurture? Give a reason for your answer.

2 Identify two factors that affect a person's ethnicity.

3 Explain how gender and ethnicity may influence a person's social development.

Family life

The experience of living as part of a family is something that most people have at some time in their lives. Many people see the family as the cornerstone of society because of the important role that it plays in a person's development. The family is said to carry out **primary socialisation**. This means that family members, especially parents, teach children the values, beliefs and skills that will prepare them for later life.

Within a family a person can have a number of different possible relationships. Relationships with parents are especially important for development, but so are those with brothers and sisters. The role of family relationships can be summarised as that of providing for, supporting and protecting an individual as they grow and develop (see the table below).

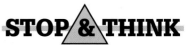

STOP & THINK

Can you think of any important lessons that your parents taught you as part of your primary socialisation?

Providing	The family provides informal education and socialisation for children. This enables children to develop attitudes, values and the rules of social behaviour. The family also provides the physical resources needed for growth and intellectual development, such as food, toys and other stimulation.
Supporting	Family relationships are an important means by which a person develops emotionally from infancy through to adulthood. Early attachment and bonding (see page 162) are important features of this. Family relationships can be a source of stability, security and a place where emotions can be safely expressed.
Protecting	Family members play a very important role in protecting the health and well being of other members through the provision of informal care and support. In particular, the family protects and nurtures the interests of children and adolescents through giving advice and guidance. Family relationships are usually very deep – a new person cannot simply replace a family member who dies or is in any way separated from the family.

Friendships

Children learn how to behave and relate to others both through their family relationships and also through developing an increasing range of friendships. A person's personality, social skills and emotional development are all shaped by their experience of friendships with others. Friendships are very important informal relationships in which social and emotional development occurs. Many important friendships are formed when people are at school. The impact of these on development is discussed in the next section on the role of education.

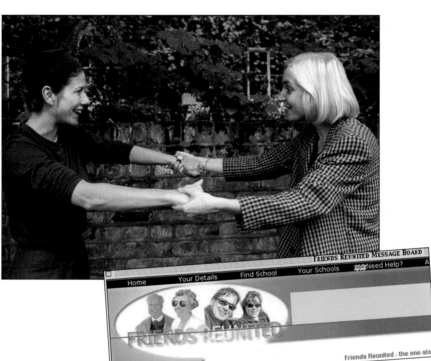

Make a list of all the current and past friendships that have influenced your personal development. Try to identify how these different friendships have affected you.

OVER TO YOU

Social, intellectual and emotional development are continuing processes. As individuals, we continue to develop and change throughout life. We've just seen how a person's family and childhood friendships play a very important role in the earlier stages of development. Other influences that are equally as important later in life include education, employment and our life experiences. All these things shape the person we become.

Educational experiences

What part does education play in a person's development? An obvious answer might be that school-based or formal education promotes intellectual development because it is about learning. Intellectual development through education results in people increasing their knowledge and thinking skills. However, education also affects social and emotional development.

In the United Kingdom most children go to school between the ages of five and 16 years to receive their formal education. The experience of going to school, and the nature of what is learnt there, tend to have a powerful effect on people's intellectual, social and emotional development. Formal education experiences are part of what is known as **secondary socialisation**.

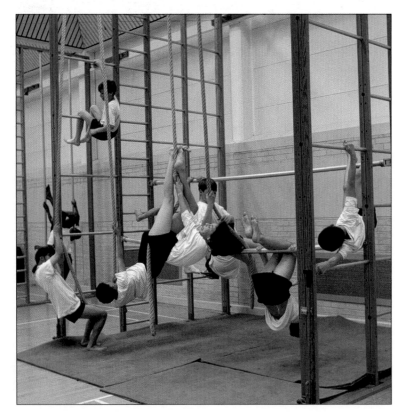

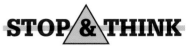

STOP & THINK

Apart from gaining more knowledge, what other 'lessons' about life and relationships do you think schools try to teach people?

Some people learn a lot at school, are successful in passing examinations and see formal education as a positive influence on their development. For example, education might be very good for a person's self-esteem and success might lead them to develop a positive self-image. However, not everybody enjoys school and not everybody succeeds. A negative experience of formal education can lead to people thinking negatively about themselves, or may lead them to develop a self-image based on being 'practical', friendly and sociable rather than 'academic'.

People in the United Kingdom spend a minimum of eleven years in primary and secondary education. During this time relationships with peers (people of the same age and social group) and teachers play a very important part in shaping the emotional and social aspects of development. Friendships are very important for development during childhood and adolescence. Friendships play a role in helping people feel they belong, are wanted and liked by others and that there are people they can turn to for support. The other side of childhood relationships, such as bullying and rejection by peers, can have a negative effect on an individual's self-esteem and identity.

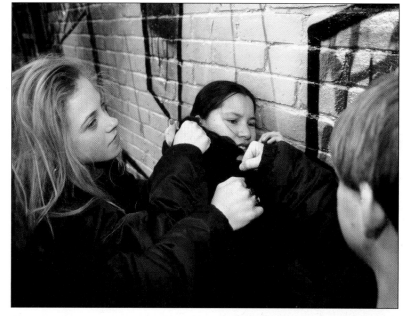

▲ Being bullied has a negative effect on a person's self-esteem

Quick Questions

1 How can education have an effect on a person's emotional development?

2 What changes as a result of intellectual development?

3 Explain how social development can be affected by school experiences.

Work, like formal education, is said to be an important contributor to secondary socialisation. People's values, beliefs and attitudes are influenced by the people they work with. Work is also an opportunity to develop new skills and extend physical, intellectual and social abilities. Not having work can also affect an individual's development. The experience of long-term unemployment can have psychological and emotional effects that reduce a person's ability to develop and use their social skills. It may also create financial pressures that influence an individual's development.

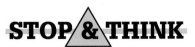

STOP & THINK

How do you think long-term unemployment could affect a person's emotional development?

Work experiences

Work relationships can have an important effect on personal – especially social – development. In work situations, people have formal and informal relationships. **Formal relationships** are those with employers, supervisors and most fellow employees. They are based on sets of rules about how people should relate to each other because of their work roles. These types of relationships can shape self-image and a person's social skills. **Informal relationships** at work are also very important. People often develop strong bonds and personal friendships with a few work colleagues, especially if they stay in the same job for a long time. As well as learning the social skills of co-operating with and supporting others, informal relationships can lead to emotional development where colleagues develop psychological bonds and a sense of belonging.

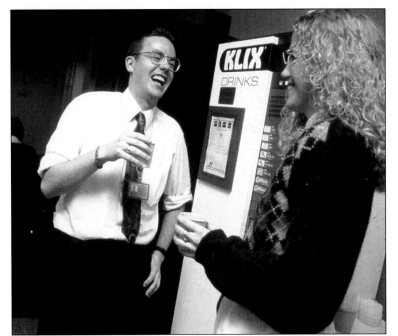

◄ People who work together often develop social and emotional bonds

Life experiences

Life experiences are major events, both expected and unexpected, which have a profound effect on the direction of a person's life or personal development. People in middle and old age are often able to look back on their lives and identify key events or experiences that caused their lives and personal development to go in a particular direction. This is much harder to do in adolescence and early adulthood as there isn't so much to look back on!

Life events are discussed in more detail on pages 208–18. At this point we should note that events and experiences such as leaving school or home, marriage and divorce, severe illness and unemployment, and the death of people close to us, have a powerful effect on our social and emotional development. Life events often cause people to think hard about themselves, what they want from life and how they relate to other people. As a result they can often trigger important phases of personal development as a person adjusts or comes to terms with the life event.

Quick Questions

1 Explain why work relationships can be an important influence on a person's emotional development.

2 Identify two relationship 'rules' that you think an employer would expect employees to obey.

3 Describe how a major life event could affect a person's social and emotional development.

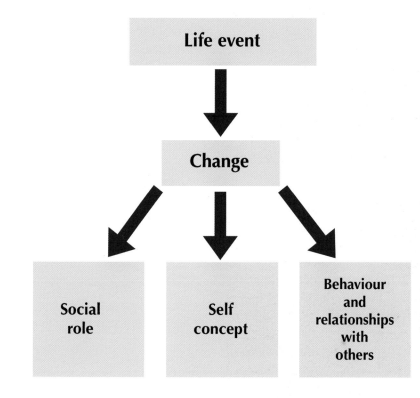

Economic influences

Personal development can be affected by a number of key money-related or **economic factors.**

Income

Income is the term given to the inflow of money that households or individuals receive. People receive money through working, pension payments, welfare benefits and other sources such as investments. Money matters in modern life! Studies show that the amount of income individuals and their families receive, and the things they spend it on, have a big impact on personal development. People who have a very low income and who experience poverty are most likely to suffer ill health, and have their opportunities for personal development restricted. The following quotation gives a good insight into the effects of poverty on a person's opportunities:

> Poverty means staying at home, often being bored, not seeing friends, not going to the cinema, not going out for a drink and not being able to take the children out for a trip or a treat or a holiday. It means coping with the stresses of managing on very little money, often for months or even years. It means having to withstand the onslaught of society's pressure to consume ...
>
> Above all, poverty takes away the building blocks to create the tools for the future – your 'life chances'. It steals away the opportunity to have a life unmarked by sickness, a decent education, a secure home and a long retirement. It stops people being able to plan ahead. It stops people being able to take control of their lives.
>
> (C. Oppenheim and L. Harker (1996)
> Poverty: The Facts, 3rd edition, Child Poverty Action Group)

Resources

People with low incomes may find that their lack of resources excludes them from the minimum acceptable way of life of the community in which they live. Because of the existence of welfare benefits, it is rare for individuals and families in the United Kingdom not to have enough income for essential food, clothing and housing. Despite this, there are still situations in which some people fall through the welfare benefits 'safety net' and live for periods of time in **absolute poverty.** This means that they find themselves without the basic means to pay for essential items such as food, clothing and housing.

Far more people in the United Kingdom live in relative poverty and experience social exclusion. **Relative poverty** means that a person is poor when compared to most other people in society.

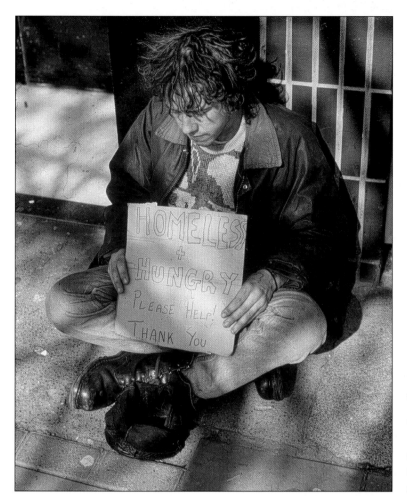

A lack of financial and other resources may mean that a person finds it difficult to take part in and enjoy the accepted way of life of the community in which he or she lives. This is known as **social exclusion**. Children born into families experiencing poverty may find this difficult to escape. They become trapped in a situation that has a powerful effect on their personal development and life chances.

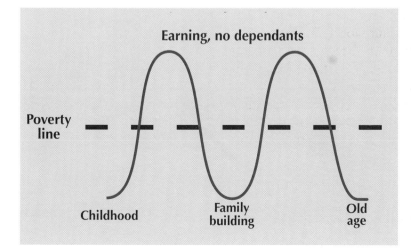

◄ An example of a poverty cycle

Quick Questions

1 Identify three possible sources of income.
2 Describe the personal and financial situation of a person who is in absolute poverty.
3 Explain how a person's income may affect their personal development.

A person's physical growth as well as other aspects of their personal development can be directly and indirectly affected by the physical conditions, or environment, in which they live. Two very important features of the physical environment that affect growth and development are the quality of a person's housing and the amount of pollution in the atmosphere where they live.

Housing and health

Housing provides people with the material or physical conditions in which they spend much of their time. The type and standard of housing that people live in is related to their income. People with low incomes are less able to afford a good standard of housing or are less able to maintain it and heat it adequately. Damp, overcrowded and neglected properties provide the sorts of conditions in which people are more likely to develop respiratory disorders and infectious diseases, such as tuberculosis and bronchitis. Poor housing can have a damaging effect on the growth and physical development of babies, children and young people in particular.

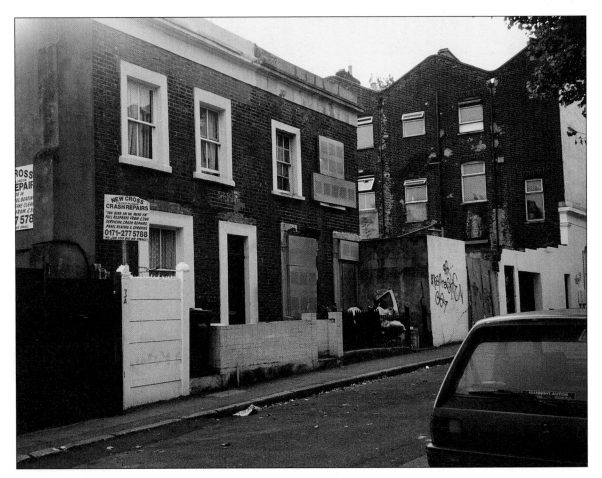

Families with very low incomes who cannot afford to own or rent their own homes are increasingly likely to experience very low standards of housing in bed and breakfast hotels and temporary accommodation. Similarly, people who are homeless and sleep rough are very prone to poor physical and mental health. They live in a very harsh physical environment and face difficulties in getting the financial and emotional support they need.

Pollution

Physical growth and development can be directly affected by the presence of pollution in the atmosphere. Carbon dioxide and other harmful gas emissions from vehicles and factories are particularly damaging to a person's respiratory system. Pollution can damage the physical health of people at all life stages. Babies and children may have their growth potential restricted and people in all life stages may experience physical health problems due to environmental pollution.

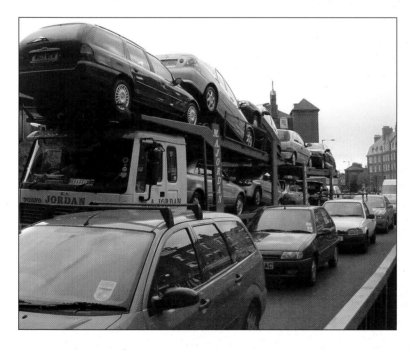

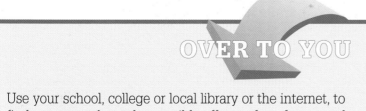

OVER TO YOU

Use your school, college or local library or the internet, to find out more about the possible effects of car fumes and factory emissions on health.

Quick Questions

1 Identify two environmental factors that affect growth and development.

2 Describe the effects that environmental pollution may have on a child's physical health.

3 Explain how income, housing and health are linked to growth and development.

1 Look at the list of human behaviours, abilities and physical attributes below. Some of them are innate (a result of nature and inheritance) while others are nurtured through the effects of the environment and learning. Use your understanding of the difference between nature and nurture to reorganise the items into separate nature and nurture lists. If you feel that an item could be the result of both nature and nurture, indicate this in a separate column and explain why.

Growing older	Caring for others	Hair colour
Growing taller	Walking	Cooking for yourself
Reading	Sleeping when tired	Body shape
Eye colour	Writing	Being sociable
Basic skin colour	Running speed	Going bald

2 Indicate next to each item on your nurture list the factors that you think influence the behaviour or ability as the person develops.

3 Compare and discuss your list with someone else in the class. Note which of the items you agree on and which you disagree on. Where you disagree, try to explain the reasons behind your choice of nature or nurture.

Build Your Learning

LEARNING POINTS

The following are the main points that you should have learnt from the previous 15 pages.

- Human growth and development are affected by a variety of nature and nurture factors.

- Differences in individual patterns of development occur because people experience and respond to the various nature and nurture factors in an individual way.

- The factors affecting growth and development can be categorised as physical, social, emotional and economic.

- The impact of the various factors on health, development and well-being result from the way they interrelate, as well as from the particular effects that each factor may have on the individual.

REVISION QUESTIONS

1 What is the difference between primary and secondary socialisation?

2 Describe the impact that poverty can have on a person's development and life opportunities.

3 Explain the role of the family in an individual's personal development.

The key question that you should be able to answer if you've understood the previous section is:

4 'What factors affect human growth and development and how can they influence an individual's health, well-being and life opportunities?'

KEY TERMS

You should know what the following terms mean:

- Nature factors (page 186)
- Nurture factors (page 187)
- Gender (page 188)
- Ethnicity (page 189)
- Primary socialisation (page 190)
- Secondary socialisation (page 192)
- Formal relationships (page 194)
- Informal relationships (page 194)
- Economic factors (page 196)
- Absolute poverty (page 196)
- Relative poverty (page 196)
- Social exclusion (page 197)

If you're not sure or want to check your understanding of a term, turn to the page number in the bracket after the word.

INVESTIGATION IDEAS

1 Use your school, college or local library to find out more about stereotyping and socialisation. Sociology books and dictionaries are a good place to start looking for information on these topics.

2 Carry out a search of the Internet for information on the effects of pollution on health and development. Summarise your findings in a brief report or article on the subject.

3 Investigate how much housing, environmental and other social conditions have changed in your local area over the last fifty years. Older people, perhaps neighbours, relatives or friends, may tell you what they think has changed. You could also look for information in the local history section of your local library.

THE SELF-CONCEPT

The creation of a self-concept is a feature of our emotional and social development. A person's self-concept is continually developing and being revised as they move through different life stages and experience different life events. Essentially, a person's **self-concept** is their view of 'who they are'.

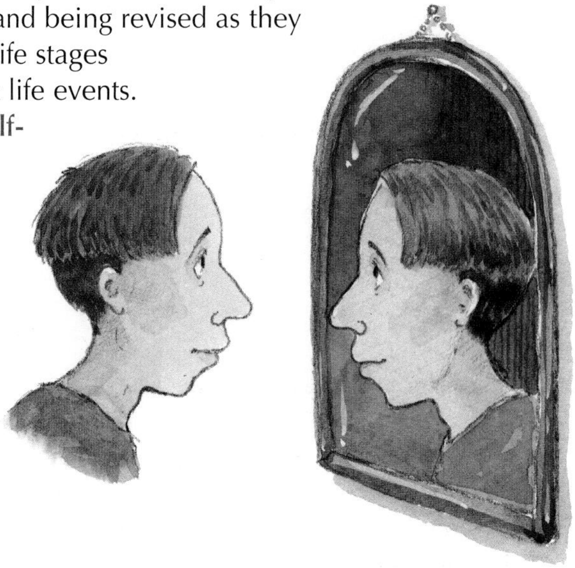

Who are you?

Self-concept is closely linked to emotional and social development. It expresses the psychological image that we have of ourselves as individuals.

OVER TO YOU

Think about your main features and characteristics. For example, consider:

- your height
- your gender
- your eye colour
- where you live
- your personality

Using both words and pictures, produce a self-portrait that describes your own view of the 'essential you' at this point in your life.

The self-portrait that you produced in the last activity describes your present **self-image**.

Your **self-esteem** results from the worth, or value that you, as a person, attribute to yourself and your skills and abilities. People who compare themselves negatively to others, who believe that they are not very good at anything, or who feel criticised, unloved and unimportant to others tend to have low self-esteem. People who are confident, but not arrogant, who accept that they have strengths and weaknesses, and who feel encouraged, loved and wanted, tend not to undervalue themselves so much. Their self-esteem is generally higher as a result.

self-image

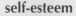
self-esteem

Self-concept

Self-image combines with self-esteem to make up the self-concept

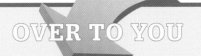

OVER TO YOU

How do you feel about yourself as a person at the moment? Write some comments about the things that you

- like about yourself
- would like to change if you could
- are good at
- feel weaker or no good at.

A person's self-concept is a central part of their identity. Having a clear, positive picture of who we are and how we feel about ourselves helps to make us feel secure and affects the way that we relate to other people.

A number of factors affect how we make decisions about what sort of person we are.

The effect of age

The image you have of yourself today will not be the self-image that you reflect on when you are, say, 40, 60 or 80 years old. The physical, intellectual and emotional changes that occur as you age and mature will change your self-concept over time. For example, a person's self-image is linked to their view of their physical capabilities. Your physical capabilities will change at different points in your life as you experience health, fitness, illness or disability. As you grow older, the value that society attaches to you as an individual will also change. In Western societies, old age is generally viewed in a negative way and older people appear to be less valued than young people. This often differs amongst members of minority ethnic groups who may value and respect older people more. The way the media portrays people of different age groups confirms this, and inevitably affects the self-concepts of many older people.

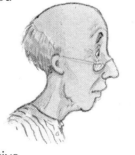

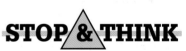

STOP & THINK

Why do you think old age has such a negative image in British society?

Quick Questions

1. Identify reasons why a person might have low self-esteem.
2. Describe the main characteristics of high self-esteem.
3. Explain, in your own words, what the term 'self-concept' means.

The effect of appearance

Appearance is a factor closely related to age when we look at influences on self-concept. People's physical characteristics, the way that they dress and their non-verbal behaviour all influence and express features of their self-concept. Again, the reaction of other people to our appearance affects our self-esteem and self-concept. Some physical characteristics are more valued in our society and evoke a more positive response than others.

How we present ourselves and how we believe others see us are important factors influencing our overall self-concept, especially for adolescents and young adults. As we get older, physical appearance and the way we present ourselves tend to have a smaller impact on our self-concept.

The effect of ethnicity

Ethnicity (see page 189) affects self-concept by influencing people's feelings of belonging and ideas about membership of different social groups. Culture and ethnic identity can give people a sense of shared values but can also lead to people being treated differently, perhaps in a discriminatory way, and thereby influences their sense of self-worth.

The effect of gender

Gender refers to the way ideas about masculinity and femininity are applied to men and women in our society (see page 188). In Western societies, there are a number of gender stereotypes associated with male and female roles and behaviour. A **stereotype** is a general or standardised idea about a type of person or thing. Stereotypes group people together as 'types', assuming that they have similar characteristics and qualities. This neglects the individual differences that exist in any group of people however similar they may appear to be. The images of men and women presented in the media express gender stereotypes and the general social expectations of men and women. Gender stereotypes do not reflect the reality of the lives of most men and women in British society. Despite this, they can still shape self-image and self-esteem in a positive way, especially where an individual is able and wishes to conform to the roles and ways of looking and behaving that the stereotypes suggest.

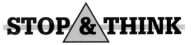

What kinds of physical appearance count as attractive in our society? Why do you think this is?

▼ Do you see the people in this picture as male or female?

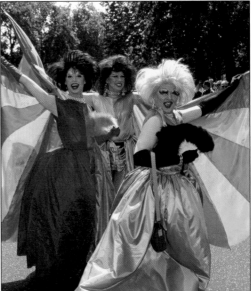

Gender stereotypes can also have a negative effect on self-concept. They can induce guilt, a sense of inadequacy and lack of self-confidence, especially where the person is unable or unwilling to match up to the stereotype of men or women in a particular situation.

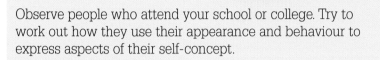

OVER TO YOU

Observe people who attend your school or college. Try to work out how they use their appearance and behaviour to express aspects of their self-concept.

The effects of environment

Housing, the amount of money a family has and the quality of the physical surroundings in which they live are all features of a person's environment. The type of environment into which we are born and develop can influence and shape our self-concept.

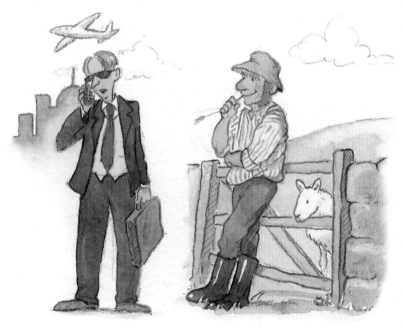

Different types of environments give people different opportunities and expose people to different pressures and influences. For example, people growing up in an urban, inner-city environment have different experiences, pressures and opportunities to those of people who grow up in rural, village surroundings. These different experiences are likely to be reflected in an individual's self-concept as they try to work out who they are in relation to the type of environment in which they live.

STOP & THINK

Do you see yourself as a 'city person' or as a 'country person'? What do these ideas mean to you?

Quick Questions

1 Identify the life stages in which physical appearance becomes a strong feature of the self-concept?

2 Describe the effects that gender stereotypes can have on the development of self-concept.

3 Explain how gender, ethnicity or appearance can affect a person's self-concept.

4 Describe how the environment in which a person grows up may affect their self-concept.

The effect of education

Educational experiences can have a major impact on people's self-concept. The things that teachers and fellow pupils say, and the way they treat us, can affect self-image and self-esteem during childhood and adolescence, when people are very open to suggestions about who and what they are. For some people, educational success helps to form a positive self-image and high self-esteem. For others, school can be a more negative experience that leaves them feeling less capable than their peers do, and with a negative view of themselves, their skills and self-worth.

The effect of relationships

The relationships people have, especially through their experience of family life, during education and at work, have a powerful effect on their self-concept. Family relationships play a critical role in shaping the self-concept. Early relationships are built on effective attachments to parents and close family members, and the sense of security and being loved that comes from these bonds. Poor family relationships can have a lasting effect on the self-concept.

During adolescence and adulthood, people go through a number of phases of emotional and sexual development as they experience friendships and more intimate relationships with non-family members. Simply because they grow older and become more emotionally mature, people adapt their outlook and behaviour to take account of their inner thoughts and feelings. For example, a young person who had a strong image of themselves as young, free and single will learn new things about themselves and have to adapt their self-concept when they form an intimate, long-term partnership or get married.

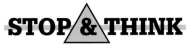

STOP & THINK

Can you think of an experience at school that had a positive effect on your self-concept?

Quick Questions

1 How can educational experiences affect the self-concept?

2 Explain how family relationships can have a positive effect on self-concept.

Build Your Learning

LEARNING POINTS

The following are the main points that you should have learnt from the previous five pages.

- Every person develops a self-concept.
- Self-concept is based on beliefs that an individual has about themselves.
- A person's self-concept is continually developing as a result of a range of factors, including age, culture and relationships with others.

KEY TERMS

You should know what the following terms mean:

- Self-image (page 202)
- Self-concept (page 202)
- Self-esteem (page 202)

If you're not sure or want to check your understanding of a term, turn to the page number in the bracket after the word.

REVISION QUESTIONS

1 Identify three influences on the development of an individual's self-esteem.

2 Describe ways that social and cultural factors influence the development of self-concept.

3 Explain how a person's relationships influence the development of their self-concept.

The key question that you should be able to answer if you've understood the previous section is:

4 'What factors influence the development of a person's self-concept?'

INVESTIGATION IDEAS

1 Carry out a review of the magazines that you buy and your favourite television programmes. How much do the images you see in the sources affect your self-image and self-esteem? Write a brief report or article that describes how the media can affect a person's self-concept. You may also want to comment on the way that media images affect your own self-image.

2 Use your knowledge and understanding of the influences on self-concept to write some survey questions that identify the ways that male and female teenagers think about themselves and develop their self-concepts. Conduct your survey by asking the questions to an equal number of boys and girls.

A **life event** is an incident or experience that has a major impact on the direction or quality of an individual's life and personal development. Every person's life changes as a result of the significant events and experiences that happen as he or she passes through each life stage. Some of the life events that shape or alter the pattern of a person's life are predictable, such as the birth of a baby. Others, such as sudden illness, are unpredictable.

Predictable life events

In Western societies, there are a number of predictable life events that are expected milestones in people's social and personal development and which occur at predictable points in the life cycle.

Starting school is one of the first predictable life events. Beginning primary school is a turning point in a child's life. It involves spending time away from their parents and introduces them to a wider circle of people and to new patterns of behaviour. For many children this predictable life event is initially difficult to deal with. It is eventually successful because of the support received from parents, brothers and sisters and teachers. At 11 years old most children change from primary to secondary school. This change can be just as difficult to adjust to as starting primary school was at a younger age.

CASE STUDY

Michelle is 11 years old. She lives in a small village with her parents and two younger brothers: Tim aged 8, and David aged 6. Her grandparents live ten miles away and are regular visitors. Michelle is about to finish primary school and to start secondary school in September. She knows everyone at her primary school. All the children come from the same village and her teachers have been there since she started. She doesn't want to leave her primary school and admits to being scared of going to secondary school, which is eight miles away. Michelle's best friend at school, Natalie, goes to swimming club with her, and belongs to the same church group. Natalie will be going to a different school in September.

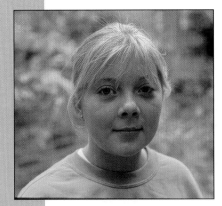

- Describe the ways in which this transition in Michelle's life might affect her in the next few months.

- What type of help and support might she need as she experiences this change in her life?

- If you were one of Michelle's parents, what would you tell her about the likely impact of changing schools on her friendship with Natalie?

Unexpected life events

Not all the major events that shape and change our lives are predictable. Life events such as serious illness, disability, divorce and bereavement can happen unexpectedly to anyone. Events such as these can have a major effect on a person's life. They may result in significant change, or a transition point. Unexpected life events are usually thought of as negative, but can sometimes lead to positive change in a person's life.

STOP & THINK

Have you experienced any unexpected life events? Think about how these might have affected your personal development.

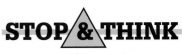
OVER TO YOU

1 Which of the following life events are predictable and which are unpredictable? Make a list of each type.

- Becoming a parent
- Starting school
- Getting married
- Getting your first job
- Being promoted
- Moving to a new house

- Leaving home
- Getting divorced
- Retiring from work
- Becoming bankrupt
- Taking exams
- The death of a loved one

- Losing your job
- Learning to read
- Being taken into care
- Winning the Lottery
- Gaining a nursing qualification

2 At what life stage are the above life events most likely to occur? Match them on the lifeline below.

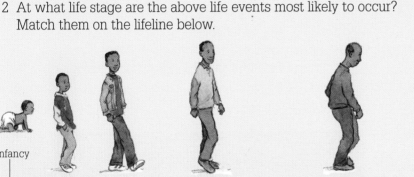

infancy					death
childhood	adolescance	adulthood	mid-life		old age
0 3	13	18	35	70	

Quick Questions

1 What is a life event? Explain this term in your own words.

2 Name three predictable life events that occur before an individual reaches adulthood.

3 Describe how a named life event could affect a person's emotional development.

Relationship changes

Relationships are very important for emotional and social development. People have different types of relationships in each of the main life stages. These include family relationships with parents, brothers, sisters and other relatives, friendships, work relationships and intimate and sexual relationships with partners in late adolescence, adulthood and old age. Changes in our relationships can occur for many reasons. They often have a big impact on our emotional and social development.

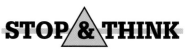

STOP & THINK

How do you think you and the other members of your family will be affected when you leave home?

Leaving home

Leaving home is a major transition in life that happens for most people in their late teens or early twenties. As young people establish more personal and financial independence from their parents, they may broaden their social relationships, find work or take up a place on an educational course in a different part of the country. They reach a point where they either choose to, or have to, leave home. For some young people this transition is the point at which they feel they have established their independence. For others, the changes that result from leaving home are not as positive. Their experiences may include loneliness, lack of support and poverty. Whether the consequences are initially positive or negative, the experience of leaving home is a major event that will always be memorable for many people.

Marriage

Marriage is a life event that is generally viewed positively and which is celebrated by thousands of people each year. It involves a major adaptation in personal relationships and behaviour for a couple. Ideally, it establishes a deeper emotional and psychological commitment between them. Marriages also alter family relationships. The roles of family members change with new members being introduced into family groups. For example, in-laws become part of a wider family network and relationships between original

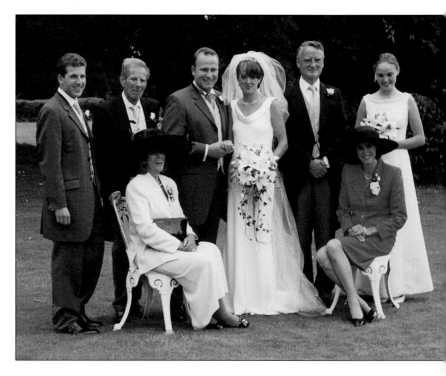

family members may weaken because of the practicalities of a son or daughter moving away to live with his or her new partner.

Divorce

Divorce is an unexpected life event. It has an impact on the couple themselves and on those who are part of a family that has resulted from the couple's marriage. People do not marry intending to get divorced, but divorce is now relatively common in the United Kingdom. The breakdown of a marriage and the process of going through a divorce have an emotional impact on the couple concerned and also have financial and practical consequences. Separation will probably mean having to find different accommodation and independent sources of income. Divorce will impact on any children from the marriage, because of new living arrangements, changing relationships and sometimes the need to adapt to step-parents.

Bereavement

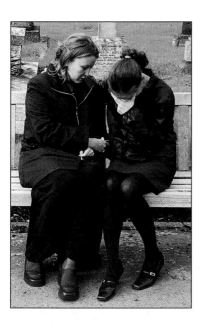

Bereavement is the term given to the deep feelings of loss that people experience when a person to whom they are emotionally attached dies or leaves their life in some other way, such as through divorce or the ending of a long-term relationship. Someone's death may be anticipated and prepared for because of their great age or because they have a terminal illness. While the loss of a loved one can be anticipated in this way, it may still be hard to accept and deal with emotionally. Bereavement may be even more traumatic and psychologically difficult when a person's death is unexpected: for example, where death is sudden or dramatic because of an accident, serious injury or suicide. A sense of bereavement can cause both short-term and long-term problems in accepting and adjusting to the loss of the person concerned.

Quick Questions

1 Name three types of relationship that have an effect on personal development.

2 Describe the emotional process that occurs when a person experiences bereavement.

3 Explain why getting married can be a major life event that strongly influences personal development.

Physical changes

So far we've looked at some of the effects that social events, such as leaving home and marriage, can have on a person's development and life opportunities. Physical changes related to natural human growth and ageing, as well as the experience of illness, can also have a major effect on development.

Puberty, menopause and ageing

Puberty is a physical process that occurs during a person's adolescent or teenage years. The physical changes that occur in puberty involve growth and the development of sexual or reproductive capability. These physical changes, and the way that other people relate to the person experiencing them, can affect the development of self-image and self-concept. For example, a person's judgement about their physique, appearance and their attractiveness to others can all contribute to the development of their self-concept. Puberty is a major life event for many people because of the massive physical and emotional changes that occur. It is a transitional stage between childhood and adulthood in which a person's life can alter radically.

Menopause is a naturally occurring physical change that happens to women in middle age. It involves the ending of their ability to have children. It is a major life event because of the psychological impact that the loss of reproductive ability can have on some women. For some people, menopause signals a transition from young adulthood into middle age and causes them to reflect deeply on past experiences and achievements as well as on their future.

Ageing is an inescapable feature of human growth and development. We all get older and we all age physically. In Western societies, many of the milestones of ageing are marked by social events. For example, reaching your eighteenth, twenty-first, fortieth or sixtieth birthday is often celebrated with a party or other special occasion.

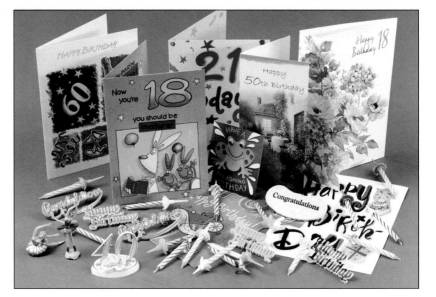

Reaching these age milestones can again feel like major life events that cause people to reflect on their past, with happiness and regret, and sometimes result in people making major changes in their life.

Serious illness

Serious illness can be a major but unexpected event in an individual's life. It can result in massive changes to the person's whole lifestyle as he or she tries to cope with the effects of the illness. People who experience serious illnesses, such as heart attacks, multiple sclerosis or cancer, may find themselves unable to carry out their usual daily routines and can find that their relationships with others change because of their illness. They may need additional practical help and emotional support from close relatives and friends and may lose some of their independence. For partners and close relatives, the person's illness may be the thing around which they organise their own time, lifestyle and relationship with the person.

Disability

Disability can be inherited and present from birth, or can be caused by accident or because of a person's lifestyle. For example, people who drink too much alcohol may acquire a disability as a result of being involved in a road traffic accident or a fight, or because of the direct effects that large amounts of alcohol have on the body.

People with disabilities must adapt their skills and lifestyle to cope with the everyday situations they face. A disability can cause practical problems, such as not being able to move, pick up and hold things or manage personal hygiene and toilet needs independently. It may also result in psychological stress and alter the person's personal relationships. Friends, family and colleagues are likely to be affected by disability. They will need to adjust their relationship with the person to take account of the disabled person's new situation.

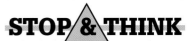

STOP & THINK

What do you think are the key age milestones in life? Which will you celebrate and which will you dread?

Quick Questions

1 How can puberty affect a person's self-concept?
2 What is the menopause?
3 Explain how acquiring a physical disability may affect a person's close relationships.

Changes in life circumstances

Changes in life circumstances usually involve **social transitions**. Some of these, such as starting work, are expected; others, such as redundancy, are unexpected. A change in life circumstances can have a big impact on a person's development because it affects the opportunities open to them.

Starting work

Starting work is a predictable life event for most people. In the United Kingdom, schooling is compulsory up to the age of 16 years, though a majority of young people don't leave school until they are older than this. Nevertheless, everybody finishes school and studying at some point in their life. Starting work places different responsibilities and expectations on people. It is a point at which young people, as workers, are required to behave more independently, without the support of parents and teachers.

Having children

Having children leads to major changes in people's lives. Parenthood involves a change in role for both partners in a relationship and introduces new personal responsibilities and financial pressures. Decisions must be made about how to bring up the child, about how the work involved should be divided and about the need to provide continuous nurturing love and financial support for the child. This can be seen to offer positive, enjoyable experiences, but can also seem a burden and create stress at times.

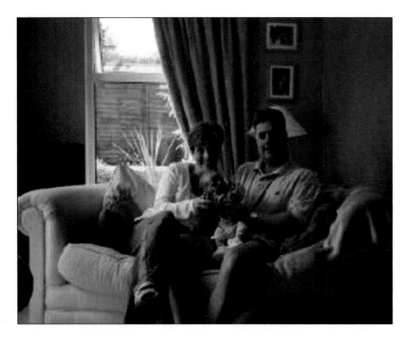

Moving home

Moving home is recognised as a stressful life event for many people. Home is usually a place that people associate with safety, security and stability in their lives. Moving home means a break with the past and perhaps with friends, neighbours and the security of familiar surroundings. The practical demands of organising the removal of possessions, arranging finance to cover the cost of moving, and perhaps buying a house or flat, add to the emotional strain associated with this life event.

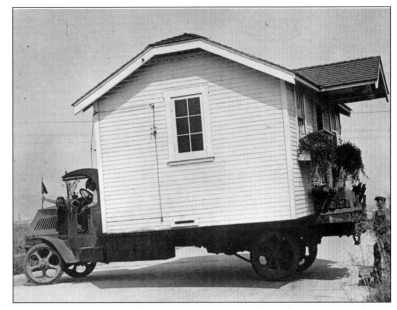

Retirement

Retirement is the point at which people end their working career. It is a major predictable change that requires an adjustment in daily routine. It also means an alteration in status and has an impact on people's social relationships and financial situation.

For people who've been very committed to their work, and whose work provided their social life, retirement can give them too much time to fill. Retirement may also cause financial problems. State and occupational pensions are likely to provide less money than a salary. For many older people retirement may be the beginning of financial hardship. For other people who've planned for their retirement and have other interests and friendships, retirement can offer new opportunities and be welcomed as a positive life event

Redundancy

Redundancy happens when an employer decides that a job is no longer required and ends the contract of employment of the person who does that job. It is different to dismissal or 'sacking', as people who are made redundant lose their jobs through no fault of their own. Because of rapid changes in the way that businesses are run and recent economic recessions, redundancy has become a much more common experience. It can have a major impact, as people lose their salary and find their financial situation suddenly insecure. It may break up firm friendships and families and leave people feeling as though they have no clear or valued role in life.

Quick Questions

1 What is the difference between retirement and redundancy?

2 Which areas of personal development are likely to be affected by the experience of redundancy?

3 Describe the impact that parenthood may have on personal development.

Sources of support

Major life events such as going to school, starting work, marriage, divorce and bereavement all involve a person experiencing change. For people to benefit from the changes that major life events bring about, they need to work out ways of coping and adapting. There are a number of common methods of managing change, including using family support and social support, and seeking professional help where necessary.

Family support

Family support is often the first form of help that people seek when they experience a major life event. Families may be able to provide practical and emotional support at times of stress, change and crisis and are the source of much informal care for people in all age groups. People need support from their families at different stages in their lives. Marriage is a major life event in which people may be supported emotionally and financially by their parents. Similarly, parenthood and bereavement are occasions when family members may need to support each other.

Social support

Social support is useful in enabling people to adapt to the personal and emotional changes that a major life event can cause. It may take the form of practical help and advice from people, such as work colleagues and friends. Voluntary workers from organisations such as the Citizens Advice Bureau, Relate (the marriage guidance agency) and MIND (the mental health charity) may also offer social support. These organisations enable people to obtain information and guidance and provide opportunities for people to talk through the different options available to them.

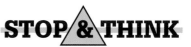

STOP & THINK

Who provides you with emotional support within your family?

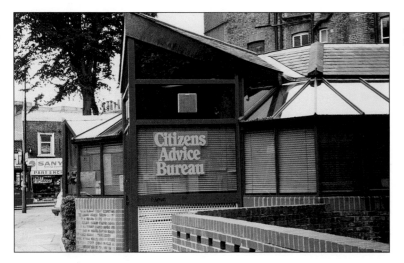

◄ Citizens Advice Bureaux provide advice and support on a wide range of social and financial problems

Professional support

Professional support can be obtained from health and social care workers who are trained and qualified to deal with the complex difficulties that families and friends are unable to help with. Where people need financial help and advice, support is available from professionally qualified advisers, banks, building societies and government departments such as the Department of Social Security.

OVER TO YOU

Our reactions to change are important as they affect our health and well being. Identify ways of coping with the changes that may result from each of the major life events listed below. Write down examples of the types of support that you might need to cope with each situation.

- The break up of a marriage or long-term relationship
- Leaving school or college with no job to go to
- Moving to a new area of the country with your family
- Being involved in a car crash
- Losing your sight
- Being promoted to a very responsible position at work
- Leaving home to go to university or to live with friends
- The birth of your first child
- Being made redundant
- Failing to get the exam grades needed to go to university or for a job

- The death of a close relative or friend
- Being diagnosed with a serious illness
- The onset of puberty
- Winning the National Lottery jackpot
- Being sent to prison
- Starting employment
- Moving from primary to secondary school
- Getting married
- Getting into serious debt
- One of your parents developing Alzheimer's disease
- Retiring from work after forty years in the same job

Discuss your ideas with a class colleague, explaining the reasons for your decisions.

Quick Questions

1 Which organisation offers support to people who are experiencing marital or relationship problems?

2 What kinds of support do family members usually offer each other?

3 When should people seek professional help and support?

1 Find a volunteer who is willing to be interviewed by you about a significant life event that they have experienced. You will need to be sensitive both in your approach to the person, to avoid pressurising them into it, and in carrying out the interview. Your volunteer could be a friend, relative or class colleague. They should be clear about the purpose of the interview and the life event that you wish to discuss before you begin.

2 You will need to compile appropriate questions and find a way of recording the information that your volunteer gives you in the interview. The main areas that you need to cover are:

- their background
- the nature of the life event
- their thoughts and feelings about the life event
- their methods of coping with the life event.

Remember to keep a copy of your questions and their answers.

3 Using the information collected in your interview, produce a case study or short report describing the life event that the person experienced, and how they coped with it. To maintain confidentiality, you may wish to change the name of your volunteer when you write about them.

Build Your Learning

LEARNING POINTS

The following are the main points that you should have learnt from the previous 11 pages.

- Expected and unexpected experiences and events can have a significant effect on an individual's personal development.

- Changes that occur in a person's life circumstances, relationships and physical development can influence personal development in numerous ways.

- Life events have a variety of effects on individuals. Different sources of support are available to help people adapt and cope with the impact of these changes.

KEY TERMS

You should know what the following terms mean:

- Life event (page 208)
- Marriage (page 210)
- Divorce (page 211)
- Bereavement (page 211)
- Puberty (page 212)
- Menopause (page 212)
- Social transitions (page 214)
- Redundancy (page 215)
- Social support (page 216)

If you're not sure or want to check your understanding of a term, turn to the page number in the bracket after the word.

REVISION QUESTIONS

1 Identify three expected life events that are also 'social transitions'.

2 Describe the possible effect that an unexpected, negative life event may have on an individual's health, well being and personal development

3 Describe the different forms of advice and support available to a person who is finding a life event difficult to cope with.

The key question that you should be able to answer if you've understood the previous section is:

4 How can life events affect an individual's personal development?

INVESTIGATION IDEAS

1 Collect newspaper and magazine stories that describe major life events that you think will have a big influence on the personal development of the people who experience the events. Write a brief comment about how you feel the life event may influence the future development of the people involved

2 Turn the list of life events in the Over to You activity on page 217 into a checklist with a tick box next to each life event. Use the checklist to conduct a survey of 10 people in your school or college. As each person to identify, in order of importance, the five life events that they feel would have the most impact on their personal development if they experienced it.

INDEX

Published by HarperCollins*Publishers* Limited
77–85 Fulham Palace Road
Hammersmith
London
W6 8JB

www.CollinsEducation.co.uk
Online support for schools and colleges

© HarperCollin*Publishers* Limited 2002
First published 2002

10 9 8 7 6 5 4 3 2 1

ISBN 0 00 713811 3

Mark Walsh asserts the moral right to be identified as the author of this work.

British Cataloguing in Publication Data
A cataloguing record for this publication is available from the British Library

Almost all the case studies in this book are factual. However, the persons, locations and subjects have been given different names to protect their identity. The accompanying images are for aesthetic purposes only and are not intended to represent or identify any existing person, location or subject. The publishers cannot accept any responsibility for any consequences resulting from this use, except as expressly provided by law.

Series commissioned by Graham Bradbury
Series design and cover by Patricia Briggs
Book design by Wendi Watson
Cover picture by Getty Images/Image Bank
Pictures researched by Thelma Gilbert
Illustrations by Bethan Matthews (except for Barking Dog Art, pages 112, 117, 130, 134, 152, 155, 161, 162, 173, 174 and Belinda Evans, pages 10, 75)
Index by Joan Dearnley
Project managed by Kay Wright
Production by Jack Murphy
Printed and bound by Scotprint, Haddington

www.fireandwater.co.uk
The book lover's website